CW00879693

Mastering your Migraine

PETER EVANS

Mastering your Migraine

FOREWORD BY

*Paul Turner, Professor of Clinical Pharmacology and
Consultant Physician, St Bartholomew's Hospital, London
and Derek R. Mullis, Director, The Migraine Trust*

GRANADA
London Toronto Sydney New York

Granada Publishing Limited
Frogmore, St Albans, Herts AL2 2NF
and
36 Golden Square, London W1R 4AH
515 Madison Avenue, New York, NY 10022, USA
117 York Street, Sydney, NSW 2000, Australia
60 International Blvd, Rexdale, Ontario, R9W 6J2, Canada
61 Beach Road, Auckland, New Zealand

Published by Granada Publishing 1978
Reprinted 1981
Reissued in paper covers 1983

Copyright © Peter Evans 1978

British Library Cataloguing in Publication Data

Evans, Peter, *1940–*
    Mastering your migraine.
    1. Migraine
    I. Title
    616.8'57   RC392

ISBN 0-246-12112-2

Printed in Great Britain by
Richard Clay (The Chaucer Press) Ltd,
Bungay, Suffolk

Granada ®
Granada Publishing ®

Contents

Foreword

Migraine is a worldwide problem with the one possible exception of tribal Africa where apparently it is unknown. When the first International Migraine Symposium was held in 1976 it was attended by 250 doctors and scientists from thirty countries.

If we can accept trepanning as evidence, the history of headache extends back 10,000 years. Skulls showing signs of trepanning – making a hole in the skull to let out evil spirits – have been found in Europe and on the American continent, particularly Mexico and Peru, dating back to the Neolithic and Bronze Ages. The openings in the European skulls were mostly oval and the edges showed signs of healing, indicating that the operation had been carried out during life and that the patient had survived for some time afterwards. Migraine was mentioned in a papyrus, written in about 1700 BC as 'a sickness of half the head'. It is very sad that over 3500 years later the causes of this most unpleasant malady have not been found.

It can be no coincidence that the increased interest by scientists has coincided with the establishing of the Migraine Trust and in the decade that has passed there have, without question, been developments that have helped the sufferers. The Trust, a registered Charity, was set up in 1965 to further research into the causes, alleviation and treatment of migraine. Although the Trust Deed permits grants to be made anywhere in the world, this has not yet been possible owing to the Trust's very limited income but the structure is there to be used whenever the money is available. It is vital that we think internationally when planning research so that the best brains in the world may be brought to bear on particular aspects of the problem.

There are many different factors that can precipitate a migraine attack, including diet, emotion, hormones and drugs. It is not surprising, therefore, that treatment can take so many forms, varying from dietary measures, relaxation and acupuncture to potent drug therapy.

The question which medical scientists involved in migraine

research are continually asking is: 'Is there one common mechanism by which all these precipitating factors produce a migraine attack?' If so, then it may be possible to develop treatment to deal with that final mechanism. There are, however, other conditions in medicine, such as diabetes, where the clinical picture is generally the same, but the causes and treatment are different, and will probably remain so.

We must, therefore, avoid a fanatical obsession to find *the* cause of migraine if, in fact, no such single cause exists.

The treatment of migraine is very much a joint operation between the family doctor and the sufferer and it is most important that he or she knows the complete medical history of the patient since there are so many factors that ultimately trigger off an attack of migraine. The complexity of the treatment becomes apparent when one sees the complete list of drugs that are in use at this time.

In the past two or three years a number of books have been published about migraine, the majority written by doctors. This one, being written by a medical journalist has the advantage that this author does not begin with any preconceived idea. This book surveys more or less the whole spectrum of present knowledge and treatment in a language suited to the non-medical sufferer.

DEREK R. MULLIS
Director, the Migraine Trust
45 Great Ormond Street, London WC1

PAUL TURNER
Professor of Clinical Pharmacology
Consultant Physician
St Bartholomew's Hospital, London

I

Problems, Problems

'There is no simple explanation for anything in medicine.'
Sir Thomas Lewis

For centuries migraine was a breeding-ground for countless misconceptions and gross misunderstanding. Today, despite the attentions of scrupulously careful, science-based research and our enhanced knowledge of all things medical, it still is. One general practitioner, when asked how many migraine patients he has will scratch his head and say, 'Well, I can't offhand think of one. But plenty of headache cases.' Another will go to the other extreme and base his diagnosis of 'migraine' purely on the existence of head pain of virtually any kind that cannot be explained by observable causal factors. Both doctors are wrong but both, in a sense, are also right. Migraine should not be ignored when it is present, but neither should it be 'treated' when it is not. The first problem for our hard-pressed family doctor is to find a workable diagnostic balance that chimes with the facts. Just what these facts are is the substance of this book.

Problem number two is that people complaining regularly of head pains and other symptoms vary a good deal in the way in which they react to their suffering. 'Migraine' is what willowy ladies in chiffon dresses have as they sink agonisingly on to a chaise-longue in some romantic novel or it is what racks a frenzied artist searching for inspiration in a movie-set garret. The factory worker or housewife, it is often assumed, just get penny-plain headaches, struggling on through the day trying to go about their work with the minimum of fuss and self-publicity. In other words, a lot of what people in general and doctors in particular know about the experience of migraine comes from a self-selected group, an articulate minority with the personal skills and resources to press for attention and get it. So who *are* the people who suffer from migraine? Intelligent, artistic perfectionists from restricted strata of society or ordinary folk with no special aptitudes to distinguish them from everyone else?

Thirdly, migraine is difficult to come to grips with because it does not conform to an 'illness' type in the sense that pneumonia or gastric ulcers do. Migraine is a symptom – or rather configuration of symptoms – that go to make up a condition. The fact that this condition is characterised by pain, bizarre visual phenomena, nausea and other physical symptoms, is proof enough that there is indeed something wrong with the body's mechanism. However, what is wrong is the body's functioning not its structure; there is no boil to lance or tumour to remove that will rid one of the migraine attack. This is something that raises a whole series of very big problems indeed. Between attacks the migraine sufferer is normal. There are no physiological abnormalities or peculiarities that can be studied and perhaps cleared up before the next attack strikes. This is not only extremely frustrating for doctors and their patients: it also runs counter to what we believe medicine is all about, the identification and treatment of observable organic illness.

It is perhaps for this reason that the misconception has arisen and persisted that the migraine sufferer's ailment is not physical, but somehow 'in the mind'. The implication here is often clear. If these mysterious headache–cum–sickness attacks come and go leaving no organic traces of their existence, do they really exist? Is the migraineur perhaps 'imagining' them and, more important, thinking them into starting up? From here it is but a short step to classifying migraine as a psychosomatic disorder exclusively, with little or no physical component other than pain. This is an understandable enough assumption in the circumstances but it is, most definitely, erroneous. For a start, the term 'imaginary pain' is meaningless. All pain, be this of a migrainous kind or the sort of sharp twinge you get if you prick your finger, is in the mind, not in the part of the body that is hurt or in the nerves that conduct impulses from it to the brain. The area of the brain that translates the nerve-carried pain signals into a conscious feeling of distress is the seat of pain. However great or slight the external stimulus, be this a bee sting or a napalm burn, pain is felt only to the extent that the brain interprets it as such. So migraine headaches are, so far as pain is concerned, just like any others, and dependent on the responsiveness of the brain to stimuli for the amount of distress they cause. This is not to say that frame of mind does not enter into things. It has been found that soldiers coming to hospital from the front line with serious injuries deny feeling pain to a greater extent than their civilian counterparts undergoing treatment for less severe injuries. In some way the soldiers' state of mind increased their resistance to pain, raising their pain threshold.

Similarly with migraine, mental or emotional factors can play a part both in helping to trigger off attacks and in determining the amount of distress they cause. The same holds true for many other conditions such as stroke and heart disorder, all of which are aggravated or extenuated by the degree of stress or arousal operating on the sufferer. But migraine sufferers are not hypochondriacs or attention seekers. Migraine may be conditioned in certain ways by the sufferer himself or herself but not actually caused by being thought about.

What does cause migraine? The fact that, basically, we do not yet know precisely why attacks begin even though we are learning a lot about how they are precipitated is the biggest problem of all. Without understanding precisely what is happening in the body, brain, arteries and blood of a patient, a doctor has to treat the symptoms, by relieving pain and trying to provide suitable advice for either tempering or preventing further attacks. To some extent it is feeling a way in the dark, looking for the light switch that may after all prove to be in another room. At the same time, new and challenging variants of the migraine syndrome are presenting themselves, such as 'Chinese restaurant headache' and 'footballers' migraine' that seem to tie in closely with dietary or occupational factors. Then there are so many variants on well-established migraine features, such as the effect of strenuous exercise, which for one unfortunate sufferer meant an acute attack directly after he had sexual intercourse! All these variations need to be looked at carefully in the context of our considerable knowledge of the body's behaviour before, during and after attacks. It is unlikely that any single one of them will throw the switch, because the cause of migraine is multi-factorial, a combination of physiological, circumstantial, emotional and neurological features conspiring in particular individuals at particular times to set off the attack mechanism.

There are many forms of headache. It is perhaps the most common complaint brought to the attention of doctors and a major source of revenue for pharmaceutical companies. Not all headaches of course are migraine. They can be caused by anxiety or tension, 'tension headaches', or by a variety of disorders such as rheumatism, fever, eye disorder or nose and throat infections, including those prevalent during the winter months. Headaches are caused by conditions like high blood pressure, anaemia and various other circulatory disorders and, most rarely, by organic diseases of the brain such as meningitis or tumours. People who have had syphilis infection get head pains to add to their other problems. Some of these headaches can be associated with migraine symptoms, especially tension headaches which may give way to migraine proper. Many of them stem from causes that are known to be unfavourable for the migraineur, such as fatigue or high alcohol levels, so there is a parallelism so far as triggering off factors are concerned. Nevertheless, migraine is a distinctive condition with its particular set of problems. Just how far doctors have progressed in overcoming them is the major theme of this book. First of all, though, a look in detail at the size and shape of the task.

2

The Migraine Experience

'When the head aches, all the limbs partake of the pains.'
Cervantes, *Don Quixote*

Migraine has been with us for a very long time. As long indeed as 2000 years at least, because the ancient Greeks certainly suffered from it and even prehistoric man may, according to medical historians drawing on the findings of archaeologists, have had his share of the condition. This makes migraine, along with epilepsy, the longest standing affliction known to doctors. The celebrated ancient Greek physician Hippocrates (from whom the modern Hippocratic Oath is derived) saw many patients with migraine as this description, written some four hundred years BC, testifies:

> Most of the time he [the patient] seemed to see something shining before him like a light, usually in part of the right eye. At the end of a moment a violent pain supervened in the right temple, then in all the head and neck, where the head is attached to the spine, and then vomiting when it becomes possible is able to direct the pain and render it more moderate.

This classic description, with its all-too-familiar sequence of symptoms, is precisely what a doctor today would instantly recognise as that of migraine, although he would not follow Hippocrates' example and give relief to the patient by bleeding, a practice which persisted for many centuries. Nor would today's doctor contemplate the treatment known to have been carried out in early times by which a hole was drilled in the skull. The theory was that the intense head-throbbing pain of migraine with its associated 'fit to burst' feelings would be assuaged by trephining the skull. Even as late as the seventeenth century this drastic surgery was being recommended though not, it might be added, always accepted.

The real 'discoverer' of migraine was not Hippocrates but Aretaeus of Cappadocia who was born around AD 80, having spent his working life in both Alexandria and Rome. He was fascinated by headaches generally and classified them into 'perpetual' (cephalea), 'habitual' (cephalgia) and 'intermittently recurring' which he described as *heterocrania*. This last, we can tell from his clinical description, is certainly migraine – unilateral headaches accompanied often by nausea, disturbances of the senses especially smell, and relieved partly by being in dark places. About fifty years after Aretaeus, Galen introduced the word 'hemicrania' or one-sided headache and it was this particular label that stuck through succeeding centuries, being progressively distorted by French writers to give the version 'megrim'. Finally, by the eighteenth century, the modern term was in common usage.

Throughout history doctors have built up a picture of migraine that is, in purely descriptive terms, virtually complete. But, of course, treatments have not always accorded with modern practice. Apart from bleeding and trephining, there are references to other methods of relieving symptoms that seem appallingly misguided by our standards today. The famous Abulcasis (AD 936–1013) used to place a hot iron against the temple or, if this failed to work, make an incision in the same place and put a piece of garlic under the broken skin.

As well as describing and treating the symptoms of migraine – though in some cases of course what they believed to be migraine could well have been other conditions, like brain tumours – these early doctors were also observing all sorts of important related factors. One early Greek physician identified certain things that could precipitate attacks, 'noises, cries, a brilliant light, drinking of wine and strong-smelling things which fill the head'. In the seventeenth century a pioneer clinical neurologist, Thomas Willis, studied migraine in a number of patients including one of his most distinguished clients, Lady Anne Conway, whom he treated for more than twenty years. Willis kept a casebook of his visits in which we find observations of such factors as eating habits and migraine attacks. One young girl had a headache one night which seemed to him to result from a 'vice of the stomach'.

Another interesting historical aspect of the migraine experience (and one that still persists today) is that many of the doctors most interested in it were themselves sufferers. One of the best known was

John Fothergill, the discoverer of diphtheria, whose particular 'vice of the stomach' was his fondness for chocolate which he blamed for triggering off his attacks. It was Fothergill who in 1778 first pointed out the peculiar visual phenomenon preceding his attacks called 'fortification figures' (teichopsia) those zigzags that resemble the battlements of a mediaeval fortress wall.

By the nineteenth century all this data had been added to by some vital observations that were to herald much of the present-day research work on migraine. These were data on the changes in the size of blood vessels in the head which were thought to cause the migrainous symptoms.

With this idea the foundations for modern migraine research were laid. The bedrock was Edward Liveing's book, published in 1873, *On Megrim Sick-Headache, and some Allied Disorders: A Contribution to the Pathology of Nerve Storms* in which he documented in the space of over 500 pages a number of important features of the condition and its symptoms. Over a century ago Liveing saw just those signs and symptoms that have been so familiar to migraine sufferers through the ages: that women are more prone than men; that the first attacks often strike early in life, frequently at puberty; that migraine attacks are triggered off sometimes by upset stomachs, menstruation and emotional upheavals; that lack of food can lead to an attack; that the times of going to sleep or waking up are particularly critical; that migraine can be triggered off in some people by over-stimulation of the senses of hearing, sight and smell; that some people become highly active mentally while others are irritable and indecisive, and that migraine is often accompanied by emotional changes, sometimes towards depression, sometimes euphoria.

In our own time these observations have been supplemented by thousands of others, and migraine has, as it were, been subdivided into many different observable forms. We have witnessed the intensification of science-based research and treatment efforts, especially in the use of drugs to combat its effects. In America, for example, Lennox very early on started using ergotamine which has since been employed very widely to relieve – though not prevent – migraine attacks. In both Britain and America scientists have made strenuous attempts to set up experimentally the mechanisms operating in the body during migrainous headaches, especially under the pioneering direction of the late Harold Wolff in New York, and there have been numerous investigations of the biochemical nature of headaches that have thrown up interesting, though not conclusive, leads. In Italy Sicuteri concentrated on the action of naturally-produced serotonin as a possible headache-making substance, coming up with an anti-serotonin agent that, while not of use in attacks, has been useful in preventing them.

So, for two thousand years and more the experience of migraine has been with us. And doctors have over the centuries identified and, more recently, carefully categorised these attacks. However, as we shall see in the next chapter, there is not even in this century an agreed, standard definition of migraine that all doctors automatically use. So how sure can we be that the physicians in history like Aretaeus or Liveing were diagnosing the condition properly? After all, they had to rely on the subjective description of their symptoms given to them by their patients and then make up their minds accordingly. The same is true today. We can read the account by Joan of Arc (a famous sufferer) of the voices which came to her, in her thirteenth year, accompanied by a light from one side and heard the day after she had fasted. From this it is easy to infer a case of migraine, as it is with other historical visionaries dazzled by strong lights which doctors have given the name of 'scotoma'. Whether or not this is the wisdom of hindsight in certain cases it is now impossible to say. But we do know that today's sufferers have a long list of distinguished forerunners: Peter the Great, Mary Tudor, the Empress Mary Louise, authors Lewis Carroll and Alexander Pope; philosophers Nietzsche and Pascal; scientists Linnaeus, Wheatstone and Herschel, and so on.

What this historical evidence, together with modern diagnostic techniques, amounts to is a large body of knowledge about migraine that enables us to draw up a 'shopping list' of types from which doctors – and their patients – are able to choose the most appropriate. The big problem, of course, is that since a headache is the dominant feature of a migraine attack, other related conditions involving headache may be falsely categorised as migrainous. At neurological out-patient units, doctors have constantly to unscramble the authentic migraines from a large range of problems caused by depression, sinus disorders and tumours, not to mention a proliferation of assorted blackouts and dizzy spells that may have, ostensibly, a migraine-like component. At any one time, too, a regular migraine sufferer may have a headache that he or she recognises as not migrainous. It appears to belong to some other category.

How many categories are there? A committee set up in America by the National Institute of Neurological Diseases and Stroke (NINDS) drew on the experiences of leading doctors to create a useful classification. Their aim was to give fellow doctors precisely the tool they needed – a means of diagnosing and treating patients' headaches through pinpointing all the conditions likely to come to their attention. The classification they produced contained not a handful but no fewer than fifteen major headache types and fourteen minor categories. In doing so, incidentally, they redefined the term 'headache' to embrace all non-painful discomforts of the head, face and upper nape of the neck on the basis that many headaches are little more than unusual sensations not head-crashing throbs. The table below summarises the committee's findings.

CHRONIC/RECURRENT HEADACHES

1. *Migraines* varying a good deal in intensity, frequency and duration. Recurrent, affecting usually one side of the head and frequently preceded by warning signs. Sufferers often lose appetite, suffer nausea and vomiting during attacks.

Also in this category are the *cluster headaches* or migrainous neuralgia which many experts believe should be kept apart.

2. *Muscle contraction or tension headaches*, sometimes called 'nervous' headaches. These are the commonest of all and have been known to go on for years.

3. *Combination migraine/tension*, the one bringing about the other, though which comes first is often difficult to ascertain.

4. *Nasal discomfort* arising from congestion and inflammation of mucous membranes – not from allergies or infection but stress – can lead to recurrent head pain.

5. *Emotionally derived headaches*, frequently from depression.

NON-RECURRENT HEADACHES

6. *Non-migrainous, vascular* headaches caused by disorders of small blood vessels brought on by flu or other infections.

7. *Traction headaches* caused by tumours and abscesses, etc.

8. *Inflammation headaches* either from some kinds of meningitis or haemorrhage or from disorders of arteries and veins.

9–13. *Various head pains* from tumours, infections, injuries to eyes, ears, nose, teeth, and so on.

14. *Neuritis headaches*, that is inflammation of nerves through injury or infection.

15. *Neuralgias such as tic douloureux,* which are localised stabbing pains owing to malfunctioning of a cranial nerve, the 'trigeminal'.

Within the 'migraine' category the big question that specialists still argue over is whether migraine should or should not include the 'cluster' headaches (so called because attacks cluster together several times daily for weeks or months then let up for long periods altogether). Cluster headache, though being, like migraine proper, of a neuro-vascular nature, is a distinctive syndrome in a number of important respects. The pain is one-sided and may affect either eye and the adjacent area of the head. But attacks are far more common in men than women, in the ratio of 9:1 (as compared with 3:2 in favour of women for migraine) and they start later in life, in one's thirties, forties or fifties. They occur far more regularly than migraine (in fact they have been called 'alarm clock headaches') coming in clusters and lasting only for about 30–60 minutes having woken the sufferer in the early morning hours. The pain does not wander as with migraine but remains localised behind one eye, which goes red and there is often congestion of the nostril on that side. Cluster headache sufferers do not suffer from upset stomachs nor do they find strong light unpleasant, while attacks are only known to be triggered off by alcohol – not the long list of precipitants that characterise migraine. According to a Research Group on Migraine and Headache set up in 1969 by the World Federation of Neurology (WFN), cluster headaches 'may' fall into the migraine category. As is so often the case with diagnosing and treating migrainous conditions, there simply is no generally accepted, cut and dried formula.

The WFN Research Group also points to other conditions that may or may not qualify as migraine. Some of these are rarely seen by doctors and therefore not easily spotted by them, but clearly their symptoms are close enough to common migraine for them to be lumped together. These conditions are defined as follows:

Ophthalmoplegic migraine. This rare condition occurs in only about one in five hundred migraine sufferers, and involves a moderately severe, one-sided headache, together with weakening or paralysis of the eye (ophthalmic) muscles. These muscular effects – drooping eyelids or double vision – may persist for days or even weeks, often for longer than the headache.

Hemiplegic migraine. This consists, like the eye-muscle migraine, of paralysis outlasting the headache, this time at one side of the body ('hemiplegia'). This may be an inherited condition.

Facial migraine (sometimes called 'lower half headache') which involves episodic pain below the level of the eyes, usually the cheek, nostril, upper gum, on one side only.

Those migraine-type conditions pointed out by the World Federation of Neurology do not exhaust the list. There is also *basilar artery migraine* which mostly affects women between adolescence and thirty-five years of age. It involves momentary loss of vision, dizziness, impaired muscular co-ordination, inability to speak properly, ringing in the ears and sometimes 'fortification' images. Between attacks the sufferer is free from all distress.

Another variant is *retinal migraine* which, as its name suggests, involves impaired vision, in one eye, followed by a headache localised to the affected eye.

So the experience of migraine or near migraine is a long and broad one, with an extensive history and many forms and variants. In Chapter 3 we shall focus on the most prevalent and commonly accepted forms, *classical migraine*, in which a headache is preceded or accompanied by short-lived neurological disturbances to one or other of the senses, and *common migraine* where the one-sided headache has no such dramatic neurological embellishments. But before considering these forms, we must note that the complexity of migraine symptoms has given rise to what doctors term 'migraine equivalents' even 'pseudo-migraine'. The latter is not migraine at all but a condition that displays more or less the same symptoms, though caused by identifiable damage to the brain. This damage can mimic the visual auras of classical migraine for years, so much so that sufferers are convinced that this is what they are prone to. In fact careful investigations, by X-ray or electroencephalography (EEG), reveal not migraine but definite brain damage. Some genuine sufferers, incidentally, often fear that their attack will actually cause permanent brain damage. There is a little, but very, very little, evidence that this may be so but the proportion of migraine sufferers at risk is so tiny as to be discounted for all practical purposes.

Far more common are the 'migraine equivalents' where the neurological disturbances of migraine are present but the headache itself is not. What can happen is this: a person may get one-sided headaches early in life, perhaps with vomiting, which later on gets added to by, say, 'fortification' visual images. Later in life, the fortification figures continue to recur but the headache component does not. Other migraine-type symptoms that come into this category, as well as visual auras, are bilious attacks, abdominal pain, diarrhoea, fever, chest pains, drowsiness, mood changes and menstrual symptoms. With conditions like these, the term 'migraine' is being stretched to its limits, as those with experience in treating them fully recognise. Dr Oliver Sacks expresses the difficulty as follows: 'Compact and clearly defined at its centre, migraine diffuses outwards until it merges with an immense surrounding field of allied phenomena.'

3

Symptoms, Common and Classical

'Lord, how my head aches! What a head have I!
It beats as it would fall in twenty pieces.'
Shakespeare, *Romeo and Juliet*

A headache is a headache is a headache. All migraine sufferers –
however they may differ as to how, why, when or where their attacks
strike them – have this central complaint in common, together with a
'general feeling of disorder' that many people are unable to describe
with any degree of accuracy. Let us begin with those headaches.

In fact many migraine sufferers are less alarmed by the headache
ingredient in their attack than by some of the other disturbances they
are likely to have as an accompaniment. Over the years people learn
how to live with recurrent head pain, often to an amazing degree.
Moreover, the headache symptom is not uncommonly met with in
association with many everyday ailments, from blocked sinuses to
hangovers. Migraine headaches are often described by sufferers as
violent throbbing pains in one temple. But the location, intensity and
quality of the pain may vary considerably. According to the im-
mensely experienced pioneer doctor, the late Harold Wolff, the *sites*
are principally those listed below. From this one can see that the
areas attacked are widespread over the whole head and neck.

temporal	and	malar region
supra orbital		upper and lower teeth
frontal		base of nose
retrobulbar		median wall of orbit
parietal		
postauricular		
occipital		
MAIN PAIN AREAS		SECONDARY PAIN AREAS

The one-sided character of the headache is, more often than not, confined to the early stages of an attack. Later on, its location becomes less specific. Usually the sufferer will find the pain starting on the same side – either left or right, sometimes this preference continues for many years. Again, this varies. It is quite common for severer pains to start on one side and milder ones on the other, and indeed for pains to change sides from one attack to the next. There are many sufferers, perhaps more than a third of all patients, whose headaches are either two-sided or diffuse right at the onset of their attacks.

Throbbers, stabbers and borers

The throbbing pains of migraine often give way to steady aching. Continued throbbing throughout an attack is relatively uncommon and is usually confined to people who push themselves into continued physical activity in the face of an attack. Certainly any movement, such as lowering the head, coughing or sneezing, tends to make things worse. Sometimes migraine pain has a kind of boring effect as if some sharp implement were being driven into the skull. Doctors are used to having all kinds of descriptions of headaches from migraine patients and the list of highly graphic terms they use grows longer by the day, from 'shooting' and 'piercing' to 'burning', 'pricking' and 'tightening', and so on *ad infinitum*.

The *intensity* of the pains is equally variable. One person will have excruciatingly violent stabs, another pains so gentle that only a sharp head movement or cough will bring them to his attention. Furthermore the pains can ebb and flow in severity, sometimes letting up for a matter of minutes, sometimes longer. When 333 patients attending the Princess Margaret Migraine Clinic in London were studied, it was found that sixty-five sufferers complained of only mild headaches, 165 said they were of 'moderate' intensity and only seventy-eight that they were severe. Rather more patients with common, as opposed to classical, migraine complained of severe attacks. This same study also looked at the location of these headaches and found that 182 were one-sided, and about half that number bilateral in location.

The last and again variable aspect of the migraine headache that doctors and patients have noted is their *duration*. Common migraine pains rarely last less than a few hours, sometimes for the rest of the day. The average lies somewhere between eight and twenty-four hours. Long though this is, a sufferer whose pains come roughly within this span is relatively lucky. Some people have to live with a headache for several days, even for more than a week. In all cases movement, bright lights and noises exacerbate – or prolong – the agony.

Nausea, vomiting and other disorders

However severe, prolonged or trifling a common migraine may be, there is more than a seven out of ten chance that it will be accompanied by some kind of nauseous or other gastro-intestinal reaction – the literal 'sick headache'. The nausea may be mild or severe, either a feeling of sickness and a repugnance towards food or retching and actual vomiting. There may also be diarrhoea and stomach pains. It is possible that the mouth increases its flow of saliva and generates an unpleasant taste a few minutes before the nausea feelings come over you. Some people use this as a warning sign to take remedial action. Nearly half of all sufferers retch or vomit as well as feel sick, but only about a fifth have the added complication of diarrhoea attacks. Constipation is also fairly common. The vomiting, while in itself unpleasant (and a drawback to absorbing some drugs), can have the happy effect of bringing to an end the whole migraine attack, but this is unfortunately not the usual story. In fact vomiting or retching on an empty stomach often has more debilitating effects on the migraine victim than a sharp headache because it drastically reduces the body's fluid levels.

One in ten adult migraine sufferers complains of abnormal bowel movement during attacks, allied to abdominal pains which can be as sharp as appendicitis (with which they are sometimes confused). If not diarrhoea, there may be constipation, particularly just before or early on in an attack. Another curious phenomenon associated with attacks is a slight weight gain owing to salt and fluid retention in the body. Urination tends to be less copious, more concentrated just before attacks, and this can even lead to the feeling that one's belt or ring is too tight for a time. These sensations are again fairly common.

Classical migraine: the visual 'aura'

The range of sensory symptoms, indeed hallucinations, that immediately precede migraine attacks are the most spectacular and distinctive feature of the migraine experience. The dazzling lights (or 'scotoma') of the so-called classical migraine aura set it apart from other forms of headache and, indeed, from common migraine. Effects like these herald attacks for something like ten per cent of all migraine sufferers. There is no doubting the intensity of these visual disturbances. They are, in some cases, seen by modern researchers to have constituted the 'visions' of various religious writers in history, as in the case of the Abbess Hildegard of Bingen, a twelfth-century nun and mystic of exceptional intellectual and expressive power. Hildegard's visions were intense, dazzling and interpreted by her as religious revelation:

> I looked and beheld a head of marvellous form of the colour of flame and red as fire; and it has a terrible human face gazing northwards in great wrath ... It had three wings of marvellous length and breadth, white as a dazzling cloud ... at times they would beat terribly and again be still.

In our own time, another woman writer, the novelist Pamela Hansford Johnson, herself a sufferer, has frequently described her own intense auras. On one occasion she puts the experience into one of her books *The Humble Creation* where her character Kate 'began to see, in the air, tiny dot and tail phantoms like germs or tadpoles, constantly dropping down out of the range of her vision and soaring up into it again ...' Some people see these visual phenomena principally in terms of their brightness or colour, some in terms of shape or movement. Others see them as combined effects. The simplest hallucinations are bright flashes or stars dancing before the eyes. These phosphenes (literally 'light shows') can move singly across the field of vision in a distinctive pattern, disappearing in a blindingly bright trail or fall in showers. They can be starkly shaped bars of light or suggestive of subtler forms, even animals, as in the words of one sufferer, 'white skunks with erect tails'. Many, many shapes and motifs have been described by migraine sufferers, frequently very elaborate and exotic, like figures from Oriental art or architecture. The rapidly moving phosphenes tend to give way to more durable, more elaborate effects called 'spectra' of which the frequently-experienced 'fortification figure' (i.e. like the battlements of a castle wall) is perhaps the best known. Some spectra strike the sufferer predominantly as *shapes*; others more as areas of *luminosity*; sometimes the two aspects are of equal weight.

When a migraine sufferer experiences a visual aura the sequence of events is often something like this: the person feels in good health and spirits when he becomes aware of 'a sudden brilliant luminosity', a bright spot on one side of his field of vision. The spot grows larger, moving slowly towards the outer reaches of the visual field and becoming almost – but not quite – blinding. The advancing edge might show the zigzag outlines of the 'fortification figure', while the more luminous parts of this scotoma have a shimmering or sparkling movement, described by one writer in the last century as similar to the effect produced 'by the rapid gyration of small water-beetles as they are seen swarming in a cluster on the surface of the water in sunshine'. The shimmering (or 'boiling' or 'trembling') luminous particles, the motions of which are as vivid as they are irregular, are sometimes called 'teichopsia' and they do in fact affect the field of vision in both eyes, even though many people wrongly believe that only one side is impaired.

Often the aura takes the form of other sorts of disturbances, as we shall see below, often in combination with the sort of scotoma just described. Doctors tend to think of the aura not as a distinct entity, but as a group of aura symptoms not necessarily all visual; sometimes two or three, sometimes as many as a dozen, all developing in unison. The sum total of the effects they produce is considerable, alarming indeed. At the same time the aura may in a curious way replace the headache element of the attack, what one doctor calls 'a headache without pain, a headache without the headache'.

More about the aura

The visual aura is a sort of hallucination, a display of lights and shapes that disappear as the migraine attack develops. Many migraine sufferers report other forms of sensory disturbance that, though not visual, are likewise hallucinatory in character.

Touch These disturbances, such as pins and needles or feelings of numbness or coldness, are the most common after visual scotomata and can be felt alongside them, before them, after them or in their absence. The pattern varies not only from patient to patient but from attack to attack in an individual. The hands, tongue and mouth are the regions most commonly affected, though occasionally the feet are, and sometimes the trunk and thighs. One or both sides of the body may experience the tingling or numbness, and the feelings will spread gradually for about twenty minutes or so. Sometimes a person will lose all feeling in the part of the body attacked. Instead of spreading out from one spot on the affected limb, pins and needles can start up in different places and spread in that way.

Movement and giddiness

From time to time a patient reports to his or her doctor a peculiar 'motor sensation', a feeling that a limb has moved or the body shifted its posture when no such movement has taken place. This is rare. Also fairly rare is muscular weakness in one part of the body. It is usually fleeting and slight though it may persist after the attack proper finishes. But it is always as well to let your doctor know about these more persistent weaknesses because there is just a possibility either that hemiplegic migraine is involved (see p. 10) or that some other neurological upset – not necessarily migraine – is at the heart of the matter.

Most common of all these motion hallucinations is giddiness. One of medicine's most renowned migraine cases, recorded by Edward Liveing a century ago, a certain 'Mr A', provided his doctor with this graphic description of his vertigo:

> His megrim seizures usually commence with blindness, and giddiness is only exceptional and slight. On one or two occasions, however, he has suffered from short attacks of intense vertigo, which have appeared to him to replace the ordinary fit. On waking one morning, before moving or rising in bed, he was alarmed to see all objects in the room revolving with extraordinary velocity from right to left in vertical circles . . . an almost exclusively visual vertigo. Lying perfectly still with closed eyes, the attack passed off in about the same time as that occupied by the blind period of his ordinary seizures.

As well as the apparent movement of objects, a migraineur will sometimes tend to fall backwards, forwards or sideways or to stumble around clumsily. Again, if the giddiness is severer than the nauseous feeling of seasickness, it should be looked at by a doctor in its own right in case it stems from some other disorder.

There is a little evidence to suggest that a few – very few – migraine sufferers are unfortunate enough to have convulsions like an epileptic fit and even to lose consciousness. What data there is on such extreme spasms is a little uncertain and most experts are not prepared to say unequivocally that this condition, though it may be preceded by a visual aura, is an atypical migraine or epilepsy with migrainous features. Epilepsy and migraine are often confused, both because of the similarity of symptoms like a visual aura or spasms and because some doctors have, since the last century, viewed them as two manifestations of a common condition. The fact that both epilepsy and migraine were treated by using bromides and phenobarbitone did not help to unscramble what are two distinct and separate illnesses. According to one well-known consultant neurologist 'Anyone treating a reasonable number of patients with migraine will not be impressed by a significant association with epilepsy or vice versa.'

Hearing and ear disorder
Disturbances of hearing and balance may affect as many as fifty per cent of migraine sufferers, a few severely but by far the greatest part only mildly. The commonest symptom is an intolerance of loud noise (or 'phonophobia') which usually comes on during the headache phase of an attack. From time to time phonophobia may occur alongside a peculiar distortion of sounds, particularly one's own or other people's voices which take on an unreal quality.

Many people complain of various noises in the head like hisses or rumbles, and it is not unusual for these to act as a warning of an impending attack. Complete deafness – other than very temporary loss of hearing – is most uncommon. Far more common are disturbances of balance, the regulatory mechanism for which is situated within the ear cavity. Usually these disturbances take the form of giddiness, in which a person or his surroundings seem to be spinning around. Like hearing difficulties these dizzy spells may either herald an attack or accompany one. And, too, they can, in a very small minority of cases, lead to more serious damage of the body's balancing mechanisms, leaving a residue of balance disorder unconnected with the migrainous headache itself.

Feelings and moods
The writer George Eliot, who suffered considerably from migraine, used to say that she felt 'dangerously well' just before her attacks. Quite placid people find themselves transformed into a state of intense euphoria, like the austere-looking middle-aged man who told his doctor that for two or three hours before his attacks he had 'an almost uncontrollable tendency to laugh or sing or whistle or dance'. Migraine sufferers who, in the normal course of their lives, tend to drive themselves hard become almost obsessionally energetic in pushing themselves through attacks, however severe. However, the commonest mood changes tend to be negative; sufferers usually feel drowsy and listless, look for rest and seclusion and become irritable.

This irritability is both their attempt to isolate themselves from the intrusions of other people and their reaction to some of the peculiar and distressing disorders discussed above. Other feelings noted by patients are hunger, restlessness, insomnia, wakefulness and emotional arousal.

There is a category of emotional and mood change that surpasses the normal level; a dramatic eruption of overwhelming feelings that occur during the course of severe auras. The physician Liveing describes these sufferers as those 'who cannot bear to think or talk of their attacks, and always refer to them with horror, which is clearly not on account of the pain they occasion.' Fear, ranging from vague alarm to severe terror, can grip migraineurs so badly that they are convinced that death and destruction are imminent. More rarely the opposite happens and the intense feelings are not morbid but rapturous. Sometimes these produce a heightened sense of fun for the 'sufferers' and an impression of apparent hysterical silliness to anyone watching them.

Perceptions, hallucinations and other phenomena

In his superbly documented book on migraine, Dr Oliver Sacks lists a number of very subtle disorders – what he calls 'alterations of Highest Integrative Function' – that may or may not form part of most migraine auras. Whether or not they are commonly experienced, they deserve mention if only to illustrate the indelibly bizarre nature of the migraine attack. Visual perception can be disarranged in some complex ways such as 'Zoom vision' (as if the eye had become a camera zoom lens), Lilliputian vision (where objects are seen smaller) and its converse, Brobdingnagian vision, and the odd fragmenting process called 'Mosaic vision' that can turn the real world temporarily into a cubist painting. Another very different symptom is that strange feeling of having seen or done a thing before (*déjà vu*) which can be associated with a host of related emotions and ideas – that time has stood still or that one is in another, mysterious world. Dreams, delirium, fever, reminiscence are all known to have coloured, temporarily, the migraine attacks of sufferers of various ages and backgrounds. Often the feelings stirred up are distinctive but hard to pinpoint, and the after-effects, in the words of one young man with particularly vivid symptoms, are of a 'let down, empty feeling, like after taking benzedrine'.

4

A Lot of it About

'We here treat of headache as a primary disease; or at least as the principal symptom. From this calamity, in the extreme, the lives of many are rendered wretched.'

William Black, 1788

Migraine sufferers constitute a silent minority. They cannot claim that their condition is either spectacular or fatal. Nor, except in a very few cases, that it interferes with their lives to such a degree that their work, leisure pursuits and general involvement in society are totally destroyed. Yet the reality of migraine is nonetheless disturbing. In Britain alone, an estimated 500,000 working days are lost annually at a cost to the Health Service of around £3 million. In America headache cures rank high on the list of revenue earners for drug companies, especially through the advertising medium of television, where at least one 'station break' per feature-length programme will contain an exhortation to add to the $400 million headache industry. However, investigations into just how many people have migraine have been difficult to set up, for several reasons.

First, there is no agreement among the medical profession on how to define migraine. One family doctor will dismiss as malingering any suggestion that a splitting headache is migrainous; another will go to the other extreme and instantly diagnose migraine without looking at other possible ailments. Unlike ingrowing toenails or German measles, migraine lends itself to subjective definitions by individual doctors whose knowledge of and, more important perhaps, sympathy with migrainous symptoms may be grossly inadequate.

Secondly, perhaps as a result of the unsatisfactory attitude of their doctors, migraine sufferers are frequently reluctant to go for treatment. The sufferer naturally baulks at being thought a hypochondriac. Or more simply, he or she considers that there is little point in asking for professional help only to receive inadequate if not amateurish treatment. So the migraine sufferer stays away from the doctor's surgery. A random sample survey carried out a few years ago showed that only about a quarter of the people carefully diagnosed as having migraine had visited their doctor because of a headache during the previous year. And no fewer than fifty per cent of the total had never consulted their doctors at all.

The third difficulty in estimating how many people are migraine sufferers is a statistical one. If it is true that, generally speaking, doctors have fairly hazy notions about the number and types of migraine sufferers who have consulted them, what about those fifty per cent who did not consult them? And, indeed, what of the rest of the ostensibly non-migrainous population? There is some reason to think that it may be fruitful to look at the general population as well as the known sufferers to determine how prevalent migraine is.

Before any start can be made, there has to be some baseline definition from which to work. Researchers have had any number to choose from, with a list stretching back over the centuries. The one that seems to find favour most frequently is that drawn up by the US Ad Hoc Committee on Classification of Headache under the Chairmanship of Dr A. P. Friedman. Their definition of migraine is: 'Recurrent attacks of headache, widely varied in intensity, frequency and duration. The attacks are commonly unilateral in onset; are usually associated with anorexia [i.e. loss of appetite] and sometimes, with nausea and vomiting; in some cases preceded by, or associated with, conspicuous sensory, motor and mood disturbances, and are often familial.'

Essentially there are three elements; one-sidedness of headache; nausea; and preceding sensory disturbances – often the flashing or zigzag visual 'aura' so well known to many sufferers. Using these criteria it has been possible to build up a reasonably clear and indeed dramatic picture, with, to date, a good deal of agreement from one country to another, even though, in the words of the World Federation of Neurology's Research Group, 'all the above characteristics are not necessarily present in each attack or in each patient'. Using admittedly fairly crude definitions like this, investigators have arrived at some eye-opening conclusions. The most obvious is that migraine probably afflicts ten per cent of the population at least, though this figure could be as low as five per cent or as high as thirty per cent, depending on the definition used and the specific sample of people looked at. In other words there are somewhere in the order of five million sufferers in Britain alone while in the US the figure is around twelve million (from a total of forty-two million Americans who suffer some kind of headache). And these figures could be substantially higher. In America, for example, the National Migraine Foundation has studied the problem and concluded that many sufferers are reluctant to admit that they have migraine in the same way that people used to avoid mentioning that they had venereal disease. They are convinced that others will not believe them or that doctors will tell them that it's all in their minds or that they are 'neurotic'.

To get round this problem, W. E. Waters carried out a number of migraine and other headache surveys that depended not on doctors' clinical assessments of whether patients had migraine but on information filled in on questionnaires. For these surveys a special form of questionnaire was devised that people could complete themselves. It made no attempt to define migraine. In fact, it recorded the experiences of everyone who had had any kind of headache during the previous year and then went on, without mentioning the word migraine, to unravel which headaches did in fact have the migrainous features listed above. One survey studied men and women between the ages of fifteen and sixty-five on the register of a general practitioner in south-west London, another focused on the staff and prisoners at a Closed Training Prison, another on a girls' grammar school, and so on. In other words, Waters was looking at both specific and random samples, in various social and intellectual groups and in different geographical locations. For the most part he got high rates of response, around ninety per cent, which implies that any results would be broadly representative.

The tables overleaf show the results of five of the surveys, broken down for men and women and young/older age groups. The uniformity between the various groups taking part in the surveys is startling. It does not seem to matter whether you live a comparatively rural life on the Scilly Isles or a noisier one surrounded by machinery and broadcast music in a biscuit factory. Migraine is a community-wide problem. The same sort of result was found in Denmark where researchers came up with a figure, based on the information supplied by 495 Danish doctors, of sixteen per cent of the population with 'migranoid headaches' – a phrase used to include possible and probable (though not definite) migraine. Generally speaking, surveys like these, using questionnaires, tend to show higher figures than those

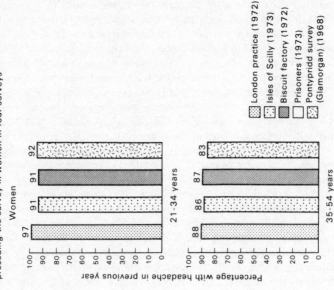

Prevalence of headache in the year immediately preceding the survey in women in four surveys

Women

21-34 years

35-54 years

Percentage with headache in previous year

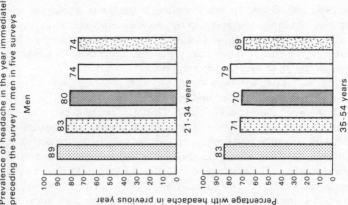

Prevalence of headache in the year immediately preceding the survey in men in five surveys

Men

21-34 years

35-54 years

Percentage with headache in previous year

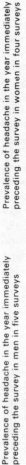

London practice (1972)
Isles of Scilly (1973)
Biscuit factory (1972)
Prisoners (1973)
Pontypridd survey
(Glamorgan) (1968)

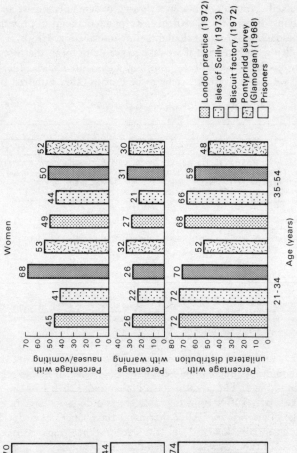

Prevalence of three migrainous features in the year immediately preceding the survey amongst women who had headache in four surveys.

Prevalence of three migrainous features in the year immediately preceding the survey amongst men who had headache in five surveys.

London practice (1972)
Isles of Scilly (1973)
Biscuit factory (1972)
Pontypridd survey (Glamorgan) (1968)
Prisoners

Source: W. E. Waters *The epidemiology of migraine,* 1974

conducted through doctors interviewing patients personally and then supplying direct clinical evidence. Respondents tend to provide general headache data rather than migraine information. However, as the table below shows, even if we take migraine to mean the three chief symptoms of one-sidedness, warning signs and nausea, the lowest figure we could arrive at seems to be four in every hundred people.

Distribution of subjects with headaches by sex , age and pattern.
(Percentage distribution shown in brackets)

Sex	Men				Women			
Pattern Age(years)	15–34	35–54	55+	All ages	15–34	35–54	55+	All ages
Headaches only	43(43)	42(42)	23(40)	108(42)	41(36)	36(28)	30(31)	107(31)
Unilateral headaches	31(31)	21(21)	12(21)	64(25)	21(18)	25(19)	19(20)	65(19)
Headaches with warning	3(3)	8(8)	8(14)	19(7)	8(7)	9(7)	3(3)	20(6)
Headaches with nausea	4(4)	8(8)	6(11)	18(7)	7(6)	13(10)	10(10)	30(9)
Unilateral headaches with warning	5(5)	7(7)	2(4)	14(5)	9(8)	7(5)	10(10)	26(8)
Unilateral headaches with nausea	3(3)	8(9)	0(0)	12(5)	10(9)	22(17)	12(13)	44(13)
Headaches with warning and nausea	4(4)	0(0)	2(4)	6(2)	6(5)	7(5)	4(4)	17(5)
Unilateral headaches with warning and nausea	6(6)	5(5)	4(7)	15(6)	13(11)	11(8)	8(8)	32(9)
Total with headaches	99(100)	100(100)	57(100)	256(100)	115(100)	130(100)	96(100)	341(100)

Source Waters W. E.   Community Studies of the Prevalence of Headache.
Headache. Vol 9 No 4 Jan 1970.

What sort of people have migraine? Well, it clearly starts early in life, though it is uncommon before the age of five. It is also relatively rare in old age. The usual pattern is this: more than half the people who regularly suffer from migraine start to do so before they reach the age of twenty-one. After that point the chances of it developing get substantially lower. If by the age of thirty you are free from migraine of the classical kind then the chances of developing it afterwards are probably six times less than they were ten years earlier. 'Common' migraine – migraine without visual, sensory or speech disturbances – more often starts in the middle years. At the Princess Margaret Clinic in London, the youngest headache patient treated was five, while the oldest was seventy-eight. The average age was almost right in the middle – thirty-six and a half years and by far the largest group were the twenty to fifty year olds. A survey in Sweden carried out on 9000 schoolchildren showed a surprisingly high figure of one in twenty-five affected by migraine by the age of twelve, many only mildly. Boys and girls suffer more or less equally, though attacks in girls, which tend to crop up just before puberty, are frequently more intense than in boys.

In adult life, women are more likely to suffer from migraine than men, in fact, nearly twice as likely and said to be around a quarter of the adult female population. The menstrual cycle appears to be partly responsible for this difference. Attacks in women seem to be most frequent in the early days of a period – and in the week directly after the period ends although the evidence for this is not crystal clear. When a number of women were studied quite recently to see if there was any pattern in the duration of their attacks and whether they occurred at specific times of the day or on regular days of the week, the answers that emerged were most intriguing. A third of all attacks started between 8 am and midday, while slightly more than that started between midday and 8 pm. This was surprising in that earlier research had suggested something quite different, that the period from 8 pm to midnight was a danger zone. Why there should be this discrepancy in experts' findings is something of a mystery. For the layman it seems as if migraine is likely to plague all the waking hours, as well as a few sleeping ones.

One especially interesting feature of attacks, for both sexes, is the time in the week they tend to occur. Married women have more migraine attacks on Saturday and Sunday – perhaps because they have the added onslaught of children at home – with a very marked fall off on Mondays. The other few days are virtually identical in numbers of attacks. Many sufferers see no weekly pattern but when there is one it tends to include an intensification at the weekend. Middle management executives report that they can stave off attacks until work pressures are relieved on Friday evenings. Then the migraines begin.

It used to be thought that migraine sufferers, whether men or women, were more intelligent than the average, and belonged predominantly to a 'brain using' group. They were, it was thought, thrusting, single-minded perfectionists who liked to be in command of the situation. They were characterised as professional people and those from the upper echelons of society (this particular idea has been around for nearly two hundred years now), all sufferers from the 'sick headache' that seemed to crop up so frequently in the upper middle class households of romantic fiction or pre-war drama. For migraine sufferers the idea of belonging to some kind of intellectual elite might have offered a shred of comfort in distress. But it has proved to be a false idea. Studies in Scandinavia, Britain and America have uncovered no differences in intelligence between migraine sufferers and the general population. What they do suggest is that more intelligent and articulate people, whether suffering from migraine or anything else, tend to use more readily the medical services around them and expect to receive treatment from those services.

There is another migraine myth, that of migraine being somehow related to social class. As recently as 1962 a study carried out by the British Council of the College of General Practitioners showed that the number of consultations with doctors decreased as you descended the rungs of the social ladder. And this tended to reinforce the long-held impression that, as with intelligence, migraine was an affliction of superior beings. In fact all it did was show, in the words of Dr Marcia Wilkinson, the Director of one of the London Migraine Clinics, that 'the clinical impression that migrainous patients who attend their doctors are . . . of a higher social class than the average is . . . true because the number of visits to a doctor for a non-lethal condition will to a certain extent depend on the money and time available.' In other words, we are dealing with a self-selected group filtered through a system that is in itself a selection process. Not surprisingly the end result is non-representative. The facts of the matter are these: there is no relationship between migraine and social class and intelligence but there *is* a tendency for more people from social classes I and II (eighty-one per cent) to consult their doctor for the condition than from social classes III, IV and V (only sixty-two per cent). The fact that specialist neurological migraine clinics see an unrepresentative sample from the referrals made to them is therefore hardly surprising.

Another misleading assumption about the frequency of migraine is that it is closely linked to an inherited susceptibility. It has been reckoned to run in families ever since Liveing suggested this was so in 1873. But though others have produced evidence to back up this conclusion, their grounds are highly suspect. Because there is no universally accepted definition of migraine, each researcher has chosen his own criteria on which to base his investigations. One criterion has often been that migraine is a familial condition. Recent work shows that, though the prevalence of migraine is higher in relatives of migraine sufferers (perhaps more than sixty per cent according to a California specialist) than in relatives of non-sufferers, it is not necessarily an inherited condition. Members of a family tend to live for a long period of their early lives in the same environment. And it may be this environment rather than any persistent genetic factor that is chiefly responsible for the existence or non-existence of migraine among them.

Migraine is a great creator of unwarranted generalisations, mostly because we do not know enough about what causes it. It might be thought that someone working indoors, using artificial light for a job involving careful manipulation and close vision, would be a natural for headaches including migraine. But once more this does not appear to be borne out by the evidence. When a group of photogravure colour retouchers working in the printing industry were closely scrutinised, it was discovered that they were no more prone to migraine than other control groups doing far less detailed work. But before this study, everyone had vehemently assumed that they were. Why was this so? Well if you suggest to someone – as had been suggested to the retouchers by a badly-worded questionnaire – that they suffer from something, they have an unerring habit of acting on that suggestion. On the other hand, some occupational groups do seem particularly vulnerable. British Members of Parliament suffer nearly three times as much as the rest of the population, in proportion to their numbers, the majority with considerable and debilitating pain. Just why this should be so is not known, but the likely effect on the efficient running of the country's affairs is clearly alarming.

Migraine incapacitates a sufferer for approximately four working days a year. This means that, at best, in the US and UK combined, millions of work days are lost to the economy, not to mention the drastically reduced efficiency of those who struggle on in office or factory. This loss of work through migraine is the equivalent to taking thousands of people out of the productive workforce of the two countries for the whole of their working lives, a fact which a report sponsored by the Migraine Trust sees as meriting especially serious interest from the medical profession and industry. They have to acknowledge that there is, undeniably, a lot of it about.

5

The Search for Causes

'... *We are standing in a dimly lit hall. We cannot see through the walls and are searching among our smaller keys to find those that will unlock the doors to the rooms. Nevertheless, we have a reasonably good idea of how the house is built.*'

Dr Edda Hanington

Medical researchers continue to have their share of obstacles to overcome. There is no rule that says that they can and must crack the biological codes making cancer or the common cold so difficult to understand and eradicate. Yet we take it for granted that in the fullness of time, these adversaries *will* yield to medical science as so many have done in the past; and that cancer will go the way of poliomyelitis or diabetes and succumb to preventive or curative measures that become freely available to every member of society. With such a track record, medicine does, of course, deserve our confidence, if not our unstinting faith. The scale of its achievement over the past fifty years is little short of breathtaking.

At the same time it is easy to forget that few of its advances have come easily. Rarely does a scientist rush out from his laboratory waving a test-tube and shouting 'Eureka' after making a sudden dramatic breakthrough. The process takes much longer and is usually the accumulation of small pieces of data, insight and evidence to form a tentative conclusion which then has to be tried and tested over a long period. It is, in short, more like piecing together a jigsaw puzzle than knocking down a coconut.

Nothing illustrates this better than migraine. We know an enormous amount about migraine so far as its symptoms are concerned. For more than a hundred years doctors have been producing vivid accounts of the cases known to them and identifying all sorts of variants of the migrainous headache, the aura and the numerous other symptoms that go to make up the characteristic attack. However, as we have added layer upon layer of knowledge of *symptoms*, our understanding of what *causes* migraine grows at a less decisive rate. A distinguished British expert Dr Macdonald Critchley, chairman of the Medical Advisory Council of the Migraine Trust, suggests that up to about thirty years ago researchers had reached something of an *impasse* in their studies. They knew enough to discard one so-called theory after another but the sum total of the established facts about the nature of migraine could be written on the back of a single postcard. He goes on drily: 'The last twenty-five years have seen a resurgence of interest into such questions as why migraine occurs: precisely what is happening during an attack: why it remits in the way it does. Today, some of those enquiries can be answered with a certain confidence, and it would now be possible to cover *two* postcards with our inventory of established data.'

What is the established data concerning the causes of migraine? Initially, we must think of migraine as having a cause, not as just happening spontaneously and out of the blue. Some sufferers tend to believe this, influenced no doubt by the excesses of pain or gloomy feelings that loom up whenever an attack starts. But, complicated though the problem is and numerous as the causative factors may be, migraine is not an affliction visited on an unfortunate minority by malicious gods. There are more tangible causes – if we can find them.

Predisposition

Everyone is prone to certain functional disturbances in their body's action, the particular disturbance depending on the person's genetically determined, inherited characteristics. Migraine sufferers, like asthmatics, have an inherent predisposition towards migrainous symptoms. This is not to say that, at birth, they are die-stamped with an inevitable future pattern of illness that will plague them for the rest of their lives. The genetic ammunition is certainly there but the gun has to be triggered off by other factors, either singly or in combination. What it does mean is that, although 'classical' migraine is roughly ten times rarer than common migraine, it runs in families to a much more marked degree. On the other hand, there is some doubt about the role of genetic factors in causing migraine, while nobody doubts the overwhelming importance of environmental triggers. So the term 'predisposition' is just what it suggests, a tendency that may be activated by any number of random outside factors. It has been suggested that migraine sufferers should think twice before marrying another sufferer or one with a family history of the disorder, but few doctors would nowadays support this suggestion. In fact, for one specialist, the idea of being dictated to by the still vague genetic argument is 'little short of monstrous'.

Some researchers have tried to typify the migraine sufferer, to find a 'migraine type' based on the cases they have been faced with. The results are amazing but not very conclusive. One researcher made the intriguing observation that, out of thirty-six patients regularly prone to migraine, nine had inverted nipples! Another concluded that migrainous women 'usually dress well and more quickly. Ninety-five per cent had a quick eager mind and much social attractiveness ... Some twenty-eight per cent were red headed and many had luxuriant hair ... These women age well.' These suggestions, along with many others such as that migrainers are unusually graceful or intelligent, have been made by serious scientists looking for a unifying genetic foundation, an hereditary 'stock factor'. By and large they have not found one.

Perhaps the last word on the subject should come from Dr Oliver Sacks who has been convinced, by his extensive clinical experience, of the futility of trying to pinpoint a genetic archetype. He finds nothing to bear out the composite picture of the average migraine sufferer as 'a hypertensive perfectionist with one inverted nipple, multiple allergies, a background of motion sickness, two-fifths of a peptic ulcer, and a first cousin with epilepsy.' In other words, people with migraine are as diverse as everyone else and the statistically-based generalisations that suggest otherwise are riddled with false assumptions.

So what does a 'predisposition' towards migraine mean in real terms? If we cannot reduce it to a specific, unified and measurable level, does it exist at all? Certainly the migraine sufferer has something in his biological make-up that renders him more liable to attacks than the non-sufferer. Just what this is is not precisely determined and, it looks very much as if it will be some time before it is, if ever. Nevertheless, now that scientists are beginning to make headway with genetic engineering experiments, transferring fragments of gene material from one organism to another – the so-called recombinant DNA research – the thought that a 'migraine gene' could be tracked down is a stirring one. For, theoretically at least, having tracked it down, it might be possible to neutralise its effects.

For all practical purposes the influence of our genes in causing migraine is of less importance than other causative factors over which doctors and their patients can hope here and now to have more control.

Blood flow – a nervous or vascular problem?

A grown man's body contains about five litres of blood, circulating within a complex system of carrier vessels – the arteries, capillaries and veins. The main carriers, the arteries, are lined with elasticated fibres and muscle to meet the demands of considerable pressure from the blood as it is pumped on its endless journey around the body. These muscles are constantly relaxing and contracting to increase or decrease blood flow – that is to change blood pressure – and regulate the distribution of blood to the various organs in the body. The brain, and the scalp, like any other organs, need their proper throughput of blood. Without it the brain would no longer receive the oxygen and sugar it requires to sustain its activities and then when it has consumed these, rid itself of the end products thus generated, such as carbon dioxide.

For a long time now the trouble-spot in migraine has seemed to be the arteries inside and outside the skull. In the early stages of an attack the blood vessels in the brain appear to narrow – a process called 'vasoconstriction' – while during the headache phase proper, these vessels open out to increase flow – 'vasodilatation'. The distinguished Australian neurologist, James W. Lance of the Prince Henry Hospital, Sydney, states that 'There is good evidence that the headache is caused by arterial dilatation, particularly of the extra-cranial arteries.' All the body's activities are intimately related to the action of the central nervous system which has been called 'an electro-chemical machine nourished by blood'. When there is an abnormality in the nervous system from whatever cause, the body, will always, in some way, react accordingly. For example, the chronic disease multiple sclerosis is the direct result of damage to the insulating myelin sheaths around nerve fibres which become unable to transmit impulses to and from the brain. It could be, and indeed is, argued that changes in the shape of blood vessels in migraine are essentially caused by a malfunctioning of a person's nervous activity, and that the typical migraine symptoms of head pain and nausea are the product of these combined nervous and vascular changes. Conversely it is possible to put the emphasis the other way round and think of migraine not as a central disease but a peripheral one. There is no doubt that calibre changes in the skull's blood vessels occur during migraine but, it is argued, perhaps these are produced not by a breakdown in the nervous or neuronal control mechanism but by substances circulating in the blood as it flows through the arteries. Is migraine a disorder of the blood vessels or of the nervous system? No one is yet quite sure whether it is neural or vascular, so a compromise description is used that, for the present at least, satisfies all parties: migraine is 'neuro-vascular'. The dilemma of which bodily function is to blame for migraine is not a new one. The great neurological pioneer, Sir William Gowers, formulated the two alternatives nearly a hundred years ago.

The mechanism observed

Migraine then is neuro-vascular in origin. It is caused, somehow, by things going wrong with the way the brain derives its nourishment (vascular changes); with the biochemical activity of the brain and nervous system; and with the electrical patterns of the brain. Other theories of cause do exist but are not taken seriously by the medical profession. Some are downright fanciful and belong to folklore rather than medicine.

The reason why these theories are rejected and the various neuro-vascular causal factors accepted is that observation and experimentation, carried out carefully and objectively, dictate that they should be. And these observations have been made where it counts, within the skull where the actual migraine mechanism operates, not outside the cranium where it does not. According to the experienced Norwegian neurologist Dr O. Sjaastad of the Rikshospitalet at the University of Oslo, these observations have tended to suggest that migraine is chiefly a 'vascular disorder' for three main reasons. First, the migraine headache is a pounding one, the pain of which increases as extra blood passes through the relevant areas of the head. Secondly, these dilated blood vessels can even be seen on the affected side of the head when an attack is at its peak. And thirdly, the headache can be reduced or even abolished by compressing these extracranial arteries on the affected side of the head. Where does this evidence come from? Initially from experiments carried out by Wolff in America which seemed to demonstrate conclusively that the pulsations of the arteries in the temple reached their height during a migraine attack. What Wolff did was to fill a rubber sphere with glycerine and enclose this in an airtight can. This 'tambour' was then pressed lightly against the temple arteries and the pulsations given off monitored by electrical instruments. High amplitudes, indicating the dilatations of the arteries, seemed at first to be the rule during migraine attacks. But when Wolff repeated the experiments later, it transpired that higher amplitudes were not only obtainable during attacks but also before them. So the dilatation theory took a severe knock, until further research proceeded to reveal that the method of monitoring the arterial changes was not altogether satisfactory. It could be that higher amplitudes did not necessarily mean dilated blood vessels and that lower amplitudes did not necessarily imply constriction. Further technical refinements to the actual methods of measuring arterial change were made, with mixed but generally positive results in favour of the vascular theory. These included using better 'tambours' and closer observation of cerebral blood flow using sophisticated experimental techniques. But still there are question marks which medical researchers have not been able to eliminate.

What is established is that the pain-sensitive parts of the head are the large vein sinuses and their tributaries from the surface of the brain; areas of the brain's covering tissue called the *dura mater*; arteries bringing blood to these areas and the base of the brain and the skin, muscles, tissues and arteries of the scalp. In a migraine attack important changes occur around those areas which fall into two distinct phases.

1. Initial (or prodromal) phases

Recent studies in Britain and Denmark show that during the aura or pre-headache period the brain's arteries constrict – a result that bears out scientifically what had been surmised by doctors for many years. Brain changes as recorded by electroencephalograms (EEG) during this phase of vasoconstriction are considerable. But there is no direct evidence on whether arterial constriction *causes* the aura in sufferers. The vasoconstriction, though widespread, is not uniform throughout the brain nor does it appear to be limited to those areas of the brain responsible for the aura. Perhaps one of the most remarkable things about these changes is that they do not appear to cause lasting harm. As one authority puts it: 'A very powerful stimulus would be required to overcome the normal regulatory mechanisms and it is remarkable that migraine could cause this to happen hundreds of times in a lifetime without producing permanent damage.' Permanent damage or not, it does herald those unwelcome headaches.

2. *The headache phase*

The first phase is then cerebral, with changes taking place in the brain's blood vessels. Then comes, after constriction, a period of dilatation when the headache sets in. This time the arteries chiefly of interest are in the scalp, though the brain too is affected. So far as the brain is concerned, the opening of the blood vessels could be a reaction to the constriction, a natural readjustment to the blood flow. This usually seems to happen during the headache phase even, curiously, with sufferers who did not suffer from a preliminary aura, which suggests that perhaps all patients get vasoconstriction but it does not necessarily produce aura symptoms.

The dilatation of scalp or extracranial arteries during the headache phase is one that has caused many a researcher to scratch his head. Is it triggered off by the brain changes of phase one? Or are the causes more peripheral? There are, as nearly always with migraine research, arguments on both sides. In one experiment carried out by Wolff, migraine sufferers were put in an ingenious contraption called the human centrifuge. This whirled them round, heads towards the centre, during migraine attacks and, as it did, the pain disappeared. Wolff took this to prove that there must be an extracranial explanation for the pain because during the operation of the centrifuge the pulsation of the bodily fluids, including blood, is diminished in the extracranial area. On the other hand, experiments have been carried out to support the theory that the brain not the scalp is at the root of the pain-producing process. A Swedish scientist, Hauge, concluded more than twenty years ago that migraine is primarily a cerebral disorder after some experiments in vertebral angiography, a technique for showing defects in blood vessels by means of X-rays. He introduced a catheter into the vertebral artery of the brain in some patients without giving them a general anaesthetic and found that they began to develop unilateral headaches and other typically migrainous symptoms such as visual disturbances and nausea. The brain, according to Hauge, caused the headaches. Many people agree with him. Many others do not.

What can be said with some certainty is that the migraine attack is associated with changes in the size of arteries both in and outside the brain. During the pre-headache stage these changes are a constriction, while the headaches are accompanied by dilatation. It is not clear whether this is a reaction of the brain to the earlier constriction or, as has been recently suggested by a German scientist, a process of 'arterio-venous shunting' whereby blood is shunted from arteries to the veins without passing through the capillary bed. Nor is it clear what the links are between blood vessel changes, circulation and migraine symptoms. The changes take place, however, and they are clearly important.

Because the changes are going on in the region of the brain, one line of investigation has been the electrical activity of the brain itself. The many millions of nerve cells making up the brain generate small electrical currents that can be monitored by EEG machines, using electrodes attached to the scalp. Although EEGs are widely used, they are still limited in their applications. Certain areas of the brain are associated with certain patterns of electrical activity and when these are disrupted a doctor can often locate the area of disturbance. But it is difficult to interpret EEGs directly and diagnose brain disorders on the strength of their readings. With migraine the EEG has been used not to diagnose the disorder but to try to establish a pattern of abnormality of brain waves of sufferers. For example when eighty-three patients with 'classical' migraine were studied using EEGs nearly half of them had a great deal of slow-wave activity between attacks, while another sample of 459 sufferers also showed a marked strain of persistent or intermittent slow activity. With epilepsy sufferers EEG readings are valuable because there is a distinctive, convulsive spike or 'wave and spike pattern' that characterises the epileptic specifically. But, so far, there has been no satisfactory definition of an EEG wave form irregularity that relates specifically to migraine, especially the more severe forms of the complaint. Obviously, during migraine, the brain must bear some form of electrical disturbance but the nature and evolution of any disruptions remain hidden within the deeper recesses of the brain or brainstem. As the search for the causes of migraine goes on, the subtle intricacies of the brain's electrical activity will continue to be probed. But, as we shall see in the next chapter, this has to be done alongside a whole battery of other research if a coherent picture is to emerge. The search for causes has so far given us a foundation on which to build. How far have we progressed with the building?

6

Body Chemistry: The Search Continued

'Those who see and observe kings, heroes and statesmen discover that they have headaches, indigestion, humours and passions, just like other people.'

Lord Chesterton, 1749

Do rats and guinea pigs get headaches? Unfortunately there is no way of knowing whether experimental animals suffer from this central symptom of the migraineur. Therefore, regrettably, it is not easy to use animals for research that will be directly of relevance in understanding the migraine mechanism. In migraine, if not in other fields of medical research, 'the proper study of mankind is Man'. What migraine researchers are faced with is one of the most intractable problems one can imagine. They know – as we saw in Chapter 5 – a good deal about the behaviour of blood vessels round the time of an attack, and a little about the activity of the brain during these same periods. But how does this connect with the body's general functioning? If that can be ascertained then perhaps migraine could be forestalled and indeed prevented.

The body is an amazingly complex organism in which layer upon layer of inter-acting processes are continuously at work. For centuries science has known about the physical processes, the movement of limbs, the action of the blood, and so on. But it is only recently that the chemistry of biological activity has been studied scientifically. The term 'biochemistry' only dates from around 1900. Nevertheless, young as biochemistry is, it has advanced very rapidly indeed in little over seventy-five years. So far as migraine is concerned, these studies have been of major importance because they allow us to situate the data on migraine that has accumulated over centuries within a scientific context. Because every single action and reaction of the human organism is associated with biochemical changes, it should, theoretically at least, be possible to take migraine and place it within its own biochemical setting.

Four common causes of migraine

In any individual sufferer, a number of contributory factors may cause migraine and we shall be looking in detail at these in a later chapter. For many sufferers one or more of the following is likely to be important: stress, hormone changes, diet, low blood sugar. Of these factors, stress, caused either by agreeably stimulating or worryingly anxious events, is the most commonly met with, though for women the hormonal changes brought about through their child-bearing years are also highly significant. Some sufferers tie their attacks in with eating or drinking certain things like chocolate and alcohol, while others find, on the contrary, that their headaches are brought on by missing meals – when their blood sugar is at a low ebb. These factors all appear to be unrelated. Yet, through looking at them as biochemical phenomena, it may be that they are all links in the same chain. According to the distinguished migraine specialist, Dr Edda Hanington of the Wellcome Trust, this is because 'diffuse as they are, all the causes produce a chain of biochemical events in the body which result in a similar end point which can precipitate an attack of migraine'.

What is this chain of biochemical events? At the most fundamental level, the body's chemistry is one that acts to take in food in the form of protein, carbohydrates and fat (alongside certain minerals and vitamins) and to break these down using biological catalysts called enzymes, ready for use by the body in all its activities. For example, one breakdown product of proteins are substances called the catecholamines, the chief of which are adrenaline and nor-adrenaline. The purpose of these amines is to prepare the body in times of danger when they are secreted by the adrenal gland into the blood-stream. The heart beats faster and more blood is pumped to the brain when the stressful or anxious moment requires it. As well as regulating heartbeat, however, adrenaline and nor-adrenaline are 'vasoactive', that is they alter the size of blood vessels. In a migraine attack we know for sure that the changes in the calibre of blood vessels is one bodily sign of the condition, so perhaps stressful situations are linked to migraine. It is a likely connection and one that seemed proven as far back as 1961 with some research done in Italy on what became known as the 'The Serotonin Theory'.

Serotonin and adrenaline

The Italian scientist Frederigo Sicuteri stirred up the whole issue of the biochemical origin of migraine when he and his team studied the composition of the urine of a number of sufferers during attacks and found an abnormally high level of a substance called 5 hydroxy indole acetic acid (5HIAA). This substance is a major breakdown product of another substance, 5 hydroxytriptamine (5HT), an amine known more commonly as serotonin.

Serotonin, like adrenaline, is vasoactive. It changes the size of blood vessels. Furthermore, subsequent experiments showed that serotonin secretion seemed to increase early in an attack – the constriction phase – and decrease during the headaches – the dilatation phase. So the serotonin theory of blood vessel regulations during the migraine seemed established, until it began to be looked at more closely. Then researchers saw that, although serotonin was somehow involved, the exact nature of its involvement was not clear. Serotonin is a chemical found in blood bound to the special clotting particles, platelets, that act to plug any breaches in the walls of blood vessels and thereby prevent bleeding. Migraine sufferers show an enhanced ability to aggregate platelets and to release serotonin from them during an attack, the so-called 'releasing factor'. However, if platelets in migraine sufferers are releasing serotonin all over the body (as experiments suggest that they are) it is still not yet clear why only the scalp and brain blood vessels appear to respond to the lowered levels of the substance.

Although the exact role of serotonin or 5HT remains obscure, one of the most effective treatments for migraine we know of is a powerful drug methysergide, which is closely related to the hallucinogenic LSD. One of methysergide's effects is to neutralise serotonin, so it is perhaps effective in migraine for that very reason. Another drug, used for research purposes, is reserpine which is injected not to prevent but actually to induce attacks. Reserpine is a releasing agent; it can liberate serotonin from the nerve endings where it is stored. When injected, subjects do indeed get headache attacks but these differ somewhat in quality from the typical migraine. So once more the facts are inconclusive. Reserpine will increase the amount of 5HIAA in the urine, lead to headaches and generally simulate a migrainous condition. However, just what 5HT's role in migraine is, remains a problem. An Australian, Dr Brian Somerville, thinks that the serotonin theory has been overstated but retains the hunch that the release of some powerful vasoactive substance into the brain's circulation is the most convincing explanation of why so many divergent factors may act to initiate migraine. We have not tracked this substance down perhaps because researchers have not been energetic or subtle enough and because they have not looked closely enough at the blood flowing through the dilated scalp arteries themselves. He speculates thus: 'It is possible that we have been standing outside the football stadium, trying to follow the course of the match by interpreting the periodic roars of the crowd.'

Blood sugar deficiency

The body is a food factory; taking in necessary products, converting them to good use and discharging waste. It needs to ensure that part of its intake can be converted to energy, which it consumes in abundance, and it does this by breaking down starch and sugar in the diet (carbohydrates) into glucose. Blood glucose levels have to be maintained somewhere in the range of 70 to 170 milligrams per hundred millilitres of blood, the actual amounts varying with how recently one has had a meal. If the level falls too low for one reason or another, the body's nerve cells get starved of vital nutrition and a disorder called hypoglycaemia or sugar deficiency is the outcome. This impairs the efficiency of the brain and produces a variety of symptoms, including discomfort, hunger, excessive perspiration and bad moods. At its extreme hypoglycaemia can cause fits and even end in death.

At the other end of the scale are the effects of too much glucose in the blood, or diabetes, which arises from the body's failure to manufacture enough insulin, a hormone that regulates the flow of glucose. Sometimes insulin is too abundant and it is this that causes the level of sugar to drop below a satisfactory one. The symptoms are feelings of faintness and dizziness and the migraine sufferer can get a headache as well, which only clears up when glucose tablets or a sweetened hot drink are taken. So there does seem to be a link here between low blood sugar levels and some migraine attacks, especially when these strike after a regular meal has been missed. Can it be said therefore that a low glucose level actually *causes* an attack?

According to the Director of the Princess Margaret Migraine Clinic, the levels of blood sugar during spontaneously occurring attacks are apparently not unduly low, a statement which other researchers have tended to bear out. When twenty known sufferers were given insulin to reduce their blood sugar levels to about a quarter of the lowest normal limits, only one had a migraine attack.

Some people skip meals and get headaches. Others, such as energetic teenagers find that they need a sweet drink before or after a strenuous game of hockey or tennis. Still others, for religious reasons, have to allow their sugar levels to drop through fasting. In all these cases migraine can seem to be the outcome. However, it is an over-simplification to relate these activities (or inactivities) directly to the attacks. An interesting investigation carried out on migraine sufferers is called the 'glucose tolerance test' in which patients are asked to fast overnight, then given a glucose drink the following morning. Their blood sugar level initially, as you might expect, rises rapidly but after a couple of hours it drops quite dramatically, sometimes to a lower level than they started out with before the extra glucose. At this point, a migraine attack can begin. What this and other research shows is that fasting or fuel-burning exercises alone do not precipitate attacks. Other factors seem to be involved. One theory contends that when sugar-producing carbohydrates are in short supply the body changes its biochemical habits and latches on to an alternative mechanism to sustain itself, what is called a 'fat metab-olism'. And this disruption of the normal processes might bring on the headaches. So blood sugar levels are implicated in the migraine experience but not, of themselves, guilty of causing it. The same seems to hold true for other biochemical phenomena.

Enzymes and monoamines

In the early 1950s some psychiatrists were becoming excited by the possibilities being opened up by a newly-developed batch of psy-choactive drugs with the daunting name of 'monoamine oxidase inhibitors', or MAOIs. These, it was found, could produce clear-cut positive results with patients suffering from depression and lift the spirits with gratifying speed. Unfortunately, the MAOIs had side-effects which became more apparent as more depressives were treated by them. Their dark moods were dispelled but in the process, physiological changes took place such as raised blood pressure and acute headaches, especially after eating certain foods. In short the MAOIs seemed to be reproducing migrainous symptoms. The drug is designed to stop the enzyme, monamine oxidase, from breaking down naturally-occurring chemicals in the body, such as adrenaline, that affect our moods. At the same time the MAOIs can combine with other substances in the body to produce unwelcome interac-tions. Because they can stop the breakdown of amines, they can disrupt the action of substances like tyramine in the liver. If too much tyramine is allowed into the bodily system through an inadequate breakdown mechanism, blood pressure goes up. And tyramine is present in cheese and other common foods, a fact which has led to a whole field of enquiry into the relationship of certain foods and migrainous symptoms. Certainly, though MAOIs have fallen from favour somewhat among psychiatrists, some depressed patients are still treated with them and they are, or should be, warned of the dangers of eating cheese and related foods.

The effects of the enzyme monoamine oxidase are also of interest in migraine studies in another context. This enzyme has a direct effect on the blood vessels; when levels are high so is blood vessel development. A large number of women taking a contraceptive pill report headaches (as well, incidentally, as depression) during certain stages in the menstrual cycle. The stages they specify are precisely those when the pill's main ingredients, the hormones oestrogen and progesterone, cause the body's glands to secrete the monoamine oxidase enzyme. So migrainous attacks here are linked to the blood vessel activity and mood changes activated by MAO and triggered off by hormones. In Chapter 9 there is a closer look at this complex biochemical process which is only just becoming clear to the scientists concerned with studying it. Certainly current research is finding data on which to speculate intelligently about the regulation and disruption of delicate bodily control mechanisms that could lead even tangentially, to migraine. At the same time it is dispelling a lot of nonsense about the alleged hysterical or malingering personalities of migraine sufferers, the majority of whom are women and therefore more prone to have to contend with a hormonal component to their suffering.

Prostaglandins

Around 1935 a Swedish scientist first identified some substances in the male sex organ, the prostate gland, which he termed 'prostaglandin'. Originally this was thought to be local to the prostate gland but subsequently several other types of prostaglandins came to light in small quantities in most bodily tissues. They are derived from the so-called 'fatty acids'. In recent years prostaglandins have received a good deal of attention from medical researchers in various fields, including migraine, though it is still not clear precisely what their functions are. Nevertheless their action on bodily tissues can be very powerful indeed. For example, they can stimulate a pregnant uterus so that women can be made to go into labour. Higher dosages can produce abortions.

Prostaglandins are freely manufactured by living organisms when tissues are subjected to a mechanical or chemical stimulus. But when certain prostaglandins are injected into people not suffering from migraine, they get headaches and flushes indistinguishable from migraine itself. Work done on experimental animals shows that if some of the monoamines (like serotonin) are introduced into their lungs, prostaglandins are released into the blood vessels leading directly to the brain. So they do seem relevant to the headache-producing process, especially when you consider that aspirin – the most widely used headache treatment of all – acts specifically to block the bodily chemical system that synthesises prostaglandins.

Thus a pattern, though still far from complete, begins to emerge, of the chemical processes in the body of the migraine sufferer acting often in concert to produce pain. Before looking at how these processes – and others – are initiated, let's look at yet another biochemical phenomenon, one that is related directly to the production of pain.

Kinins

If you drain off the fluid that surrounds a blister and cut away the skin, a raw, tender area is exposed. Then if the fluid, which previously protected this raw area, is dropped back on it an hour later, the area becomes very painful. Something must have happened to the fluid as it lay in its test-tube to make it sting whereas before it soothed. What happened in fact was a chemical reaction in the fluid during which a pain-producing substance called bradykinin is made. Pure bradykinin, even in minute quantities, will cause pain in various ways, including intense headaches when injected into the carotid artery (the main blood supply route from the heart to the brain). Sometimes this pain is accompanied by visual disturbances and nausea of a distinctly migrainous kind. Even smaller dosages of bradykinin produce not pain but dilated blood vessels which could be of relevance in migraine attacks and a tendency to permeability in the sides of these vessels, thereby allowing any substances in them to filter through to the surrounding tissue. Because the fluid plasma of normal blood contains numbers of kinins, some of which can produce pain, the implications of this are clear. Kinins, though we know as yet relatively little about them, may also be an agent in migraine, another contributory factor in a biochemical process most strongly characterised by a disturbance of the body's amine metabolism.

7

Pulling the Triggers

'. . . a permanent pain of the head, liable to be increased by noises, cries, a brilliant light, drinking of wine or strong smelling things which fill the head . . .'

Paulus Aegineta, sixth century AD

Although many migraine sufferers feel as if their attacks are an unshakeable curse, liable to bite when their defences are at their lowest ebb, the overwhelmingly consensus of opinion among medical experts is that when the symptom-producing mechanism gets under way it is because something has triggered it off. But it is not easy to identify precisely what that something is. According to Dr Katherina Dalton, of the Department of Psychological Medicine at London's University College Hospital, 'the trigger factor is too often masked by a false and apparently obvious cause, so the physician must interrogate, cross-examine and sift all available evidence if he is to isolate the specific causative factor in each patient'. Furthermore, the doctor has a number of possible candidates to choose from. Moreover, *individual* factors may not produce migraine symptoms while *combinations* will. The combination will in addition vary from person to person. Isolating these precipitating factors is a difficult as well as important problem but it is one that the sufferer himself can greatly help to solve.

The variety of triggers

From many hundreds of case records it is possible to compile a long and varied list of factors provoking attacks, coming under the broad headings of:

* Dietary
* Hormonal
* Psychological and emotional
* Physical
* Environmental

It is well known that eating habits play some part in migraine. In fact, since food is the body's fuel, it is hardly surprising that this should be so. Certain foods are widely recognised key offenders: cheese and other dairy produce, chocolate, citrus fruits, fried foods and alcohol being the ones most often specified, while skipping meals or prolonged dieting can also bring on attacks. Hormonal factors, such as low blood sugar, the contraceptive pill and menstrual periods are also frequently specified, as are stressful situations, excitement or worry. Physical stress, especially over-exertion, can trigger off an attack, but so can a change of work routine such as you might make with a new job or shift work. Then there are a whole host of environmental factors ranging from those that can to some extent be controlled (such as sleeping in late or watching the flicker of TV or movies) to those that cannot, such as weather and climatic conditions. In this category come triggers such as bright, glaring light, powerful smells, and loud noises. It is a category that shows much individual variation. For example, a lie-in until eleven o'clock on a Sunday morning might be as powerful a precipitant for one person as too little sleep for another.

Obviously many of these factors can occur in combination, some of which can be instrumental in stimulating attacks. Travelling a long distance on a train with inadequate buffet arrangements just before a menstrual period brings together a clutch of factors that cumulatively could provoke an attack. Knowing whether it will or not is an important skill for the sufferer who wants to keep clear of trouble. The problem is: How can one know?

It is easier to know in some cases than in others. During the explorer Scott's final, fatal expedition to the Antarctic his medical officer, Edward Wilson, kept a diary that showed that he too was a migraine sufferer. He was, moreover, able to use his attacks almost as a meteorological forecast because they always came on about twelve hours before the onset of a blizzard. At the Birmingham Migraine Clinic, two researchers, Harding and Debney, studied the sensitivity of migraine patients to flickering lights and found that 'the most evocative visual precipitants for migraine attacks are fluorescent lights, car headlights, direct or interrupted bright sunlight and striped patterns'. Some people have certain cells in the brain that are more excitable than normal in response to light, especially intermittent flashes at the rate of fourteen to sixteen per second. And a large proportion of these people have been shown to suffer from migraine, so it is not difficult to establish, in some degree at least, that repeated flashes of sunlight on water, say, or on snow triggered off their attacks. For sufferers of this kind, not surprisingly, polaroid sunglasses are an indispensable item in the holiday travel bag.

Another common, environmental, precipitant of migraine attacks is a dry, dust-laden atmosphere. Under dry conditions electrically-charged dust particles in the air are breathed into the body and cause certain chemical substances to be released that may constrict blood vessels and trigger off the migraine response. One electrical engineer has made a study of the effects of electric and magnetic forces on organic processes and concluded that, for certain susceptible people, they are considerable. He attributes this to the flow of 'positive ions' into the body and cites the example of the warm dry winds in the Middle East that blow in from the desert affecting many people with a host of symptoms, including migrainous ones. Why this should be so is perhaps explicable by the fact that positive ions appear to increase serotonin levels, which could account for the migrainous component of the attacks.

On the other hand, though bright or dry surrounding conditions may be related fairly directly to an attack (though not conclusively, as usually they crop up in association with other possible triggering factors), there is more doubt about cold conditions. Some sufferers report the onset of migraine after a cold bathe and for some time this was assumed to be the direct result of chilling body temperatures. However, a recent piece of research failed to support this assumption. So if a migraine attack seems to come after a visit to the local swimming baths, perhaps the precipitant is not the cold water but the noise of fellow bathers or the tiresome effort involved in getting through the traffic to reach the pool in the first place.

The British Migraine Trust has collected together many of, if not all, the precipitating factors for migraine, into a 'Trigger Check List' which is reproduced at the end of this chapter. Depending on how you count the items it contains, the range of triggers is over thirty, many of which could be acting in combination to produce an attack. So how can the sufferer hope to isolate the factors operating in his, or more likely her, particular instance? The only way is to do what Dr Katherina Dalton did for her patients and keep a record of each attack using a 'Frequency Chart' and an 'Attack Form'.

The Frequency Chart can look something like this:

Attack	Jan.	Feb.	Mar.	April	May	June	July	Aug.	Sept.	Oct.	Nov.	Dec.
1												
2												
3												
4												
5												
6												

etc.

Each time an attack occurs it is marked with a tick in the appropriate box. Women should indicate, say, with a letter 'M', if, at the time of an attack, a menstrual period is under way. If attacks seem to be occurring on the same day or days of the week then a note of these should be made *at the time of the attack*. The 'Attack Forms' are given by Dr Dalton to sufferers immediately after they have got over an attack and record, quite simply:

> Time of Day
> Duration
> Days before next menstruation
> Stress or anxiety before the attack
> Activity or tiredness before the attack
> Food eaten for all meals, and when

This information, together with the frequency data, can if interpreted properly be highly useful in selecting those trigger factors likely to be operating in a particular case. However, it is not always easy to interpret this information without further thought about the circumstances that gave rise to it. For example, attacks on waking in the morning are a common occurrence, the most obvious cause being hunger, i.e. low blood sugar. Yet a psychological or emotional element (see Chapter 10) may enter in as well which is less obvious, such as the feelings of frustration occasioned by unsatisfactory sexual activity the day or night before. Another example might be an attack apparently triggered off by a long journey to see a relative. Was it the travelling that was responsible or the argument with the relative at the other end?

In later chapters we shall be looking in greater detail at specific triggers and the first steps in a self-help approach to treating migraine – by eliminating them. But before attempting treatment, you must know what it is you are dealing with, so, if you suffer from migraine, it will help you and your doctor to put down as they happen all the salient features of every attack.

Trigger Check List

Anxiety
Worry
Emotion
Depression
Shock
Excitement
Over-exertion
Physical or mental fatigue
Bending or stooping (e.g. gardening)
Lifting weights or straining
Change of routine (holidays, shiftwork)
Late rising, especially weekends
Travel
Change of climate or weather
High winds
Bright lights and glare

Prolonged TV watching
Very hot baths
Noise
Intense smells
Certain foods, e.g. fried foods, chocolate, citrus fruits, cheese, pastry
Sleeping tablets
Alcohol
Lack of food
Irregular meals
Menstruation
Menopause
High blood pressure
Oral contraceptives
Toothache and other local head or neck pains

Deliberate attacks

No one would choose to trigger off a migraine attack – except doctors who, if they could do so, might be one step nearer to controlling these precipitating factors. So far migraine research has had relatively little success in producing typical attacks at will, though it has had some positive results. At Britain's National Hospital for Nervous Diseases, two doctors, Blau and Cumings, decided to investigate the action of fasting on twelve people (two were patients, ten volunteers) all of whom were migraine sufferers. The researchers reasoned that, because some patients appeared to develop migrainous headaches after missing meals, perhaps deliberate food deprivation would produce similar effects by lowering the body's blood sugars. They chose two days for their experiment. On the first, the twelve subjects all ate and drank normally while, on the second, no food had been taken (a few warm drinks were allowed) after 10 pm the evening before. During both days blood sugar levels were frequently measured. The results were interesting. On the 'normal' day not one of the twelve developed a headache. However, on the fasting day no fewer than six did have migraine attacks which began usually between 9 am and 12 noon. In some cases headaches developed into throbbing pains accompanied by nausea, vomiting and other sensory symptoms. This does not mean that the six people who had these attacks might always have them as a result of missing meals, but it does, in their case, suggest that they should put this trigger high on their personal list of precipitating factors.

8

The Proof of the Pudding

*'Melted butter, fat meats, spices, meat-pies, hot buttered toast,
and malt liquors when strong and hoppy ...'*
John Fothergill

Advice about what foods we should eat and what we should avoid is
easy to come by. Food experts are perhaps thicker on the ground
than many other species of pundits, chiefly because whatever they
say, sense or nonsense, people in general will listen to them. After all,
food, as well as being a fundamental biological necessity, is an important personal activity in other ways. It determines the curve (or
bulge) of our waistlines, and our ability or otherwise to run cheer-
fully up a flight of stairs. It provides a social focal point, whether in
the home or restaurant, and a chance to bask in the individualistic
pleasure of indulging one's taste. Eating is, in short, an intimate
activity shared by all, a common need fulfilled at the most personal
level. Conversely, as action breeds reaction, so food and drink affect
different people in different ways; not just in terms of tickling the
palate or alienating it, but in more straightforward physiological
terms. Some foods simply do not agree with us and our bodies. So far
as migraines are concerned, research has shown that between one-
quarter and one-third of migraine sufferers are definitely 'food sensitive'.

Allergy or not?
Food allergies are many and varied. Some people's skin reacts to
their eating strawberries by coming out in a rash; others will, without
fail, get an upset stomach from eating shellfish. What is happening in
such situations is that, by eating strawberries or crab, these people
are setting up a peculiar sort of reaction in their bodies, a reaction
that is usually reserved for harmful chemical intruders. They are

forming antibodies not against infection but against innocent every-day items of food. It may not be just food; thousands of things can stimulate allergic responses, from cat's fur to dandelion leaves.

This poses one obvious question. If migraine seems to be triggered off by eating chocolate pudding in the same way as a neck rash might be, are the headaches and other symptoms effectively an allergic reaction? For many years this was believed to be so. In fact many people now, patients and doctors, still believe it to be the case, an assumption supported by the high rate of allergic reactions of various kinds among migraine sufferers. Their headaches seem to be another manifestation of their other experiences of allergy.

Migraine and allergies are certainly similar in a number of ways, but are basically different in their biological nature since an allergy is a localised cellular sensitivity while migraine is a rather more complex, cerebral response. The fact that they appear to co-exist to a high degree (in a study of forty-six migraineurs more than a third had allergies of one kind or another) and indeed, as has also been shown, that active allergies can 'lower the threshold' as it were to migraine, is a red herring. Migraine is not an allergy though, like allergy, it is perhaps a difficulty in adaptation of the body to various stimuli, one of which could be food.

Food, humours and headaches

Until the end of the eighteenth century the whole of medical thinking had been dominated by two general theories that, though subsequently overtaken by scientific medicine still persist in fragmentary form. These antiquated ideas, the theory of humours and the 'sympathetic' theory, vied with each other for the support of doctors, some of whom managed to subscribe to both simultaneously. The sympathetic theories were of a quasi-religious nature. In the case of migraine it was thought that the sick headache originated in an organ such as the bowel or the womb but got sent around the body by a peculiar form of communication – called 'sympathy'. The humoral theory was equally colourful. The body was thought to be permeated by four fluids, corresponding to the four elements believed to make up the matter of the universe. The humours, black bile (earth), blood (air), yellow bile (fire), and phlegm (water), dictated both a person's temperament – thus the term 'phlegmatic' for a sluggish disposition – and his or her state of health. Migraine was thought to be caused by 'a superfluity of bilious humour', and the sufferer had to have this drawn off or purged by various emetics, laxatives, cathartics or purgatives. Although the humoral theory is, to the modern mind, a relic of a 'pre-scientific' age of medical thinking, some of its implications are still with us, and in an intriguing way. The humoral approach suggested that fatty foods drew bilious humours to the stomach so that the migraine sufferer should avoid them and keep to a rather plain diet – reasonable advice to today's sufferer also. Also, the retention of humours by constipation, the accumulation of them in the liver and the concentration of them in the blood, all stimulated mediaeval therapies that have echoes today. Constipation is often still considered to provoke or at least herald an attack, while 'liver pills' are still sometimes recommended to combat the sick headache. Most interesting of all is the fact that high blood concentrations of black bile were, in the sixteenth and seventeenth centuries, frequently treated by blood letting. Mercifully, we do not still have leeches stuck to us by doctors today but, as we saw in Chapter 5, some of the most up-to-date biochemical research does concentrate precisely on the blood and its composition. In the words of Oliver Sacks: 'It is not, perhaps, unduly far-fetched to regard current chemical theories of the origin of migraine as intellectual descendants of the ancient humoral doctrines.'

Which foods are the culprits?

For some people, certain foods can trigger off a migraine attack. This does not make these foods a fundamental *cause* of migraine. We do not know what causes the particular susceptibility of the migraineur, only what biochemical and vascular mechanisms are implicated in a typical attack. Diet must therefore be thought of only as a provocative factor, but an important one, for the simple reason that, with thought and care, it is a factor that we can modify and control.

Dr Edda Hanington decided to try to produce a league table of those foods that are commonly associated with migraine attacks. To do so she exploited the knowledge and experience of sufferers themselves, very many of whom over the years learn to spot offending foods and avoid them. After collecting comments from five hundred migrainous subjects, she drew up a list of foods and the proportions of her respondents who avoided them because they regarded them as migraine precipitants. The results were as follows:

Dietary precipitant	Rate of avoidance
	%
Chocolate	74
Cheese and dairy products	47
Fruit esp. citrus fruits	30
Alcohol	25
Fried fatty foods	18
Vegetables	18
Tea/coffee	15
Meat (pork in particular)	14
Seafood	10

The tyrant tyramine, and others

Having established the most prevalent migraine-linked foods, Dr Hanington's next task was to look for a common ingredient, something that might act perhaps on the blood vessels in the head to cause headache. She observed that these foods also occasionally brought on severe headaches and high blood pressure in *non*-migraine sufferers undergoing a particular drug therapy for depression. The drugs being given to them were the so-called monoamine oxidase inhibitors (MOAIs) which block the breakdown (and so increase the concentration) of amines like adrenaline and nor-adrenaline in the body. Psychiatrists can use the MOAIs to raise the spirits but ever since they began to introduce them into treatment these side-effects of headache and hypertension became apparent. Some side-effects were more serious than this and even, in a few cases, fatal. What caused the headaches in depressed patients and what was the link with migraine? The answer was a substance contained in cheese, Marmite and other foods, called tyramine – an amine, usually broken down in the liver, that regulates blood pressure. Tyramine, it seemed, was being introduced into a body that could not adapt to it. To test the theory Dr Hanington gave an experimental dose of 125 mg. of tyramine in capsule form to fifty migraine patients who regularly reported dietary precipitating factors and a dummy control capsule containing lactose that, though inert, looked identical to the tyramine. Her results were overwhelmingly in favour of the tyramine hypothesis. The rate of attack (see below) was consistently high when tyramine was administered, and these attacks came on within twenty-four hours.

Tyramine was then seen as the villain of the piece, but there was one problem. Chocolate, the trigger in three-quarters of the dietary migraine sufferers questioned, contains very little or no tyramine. So what now? The constituents of chocolate were analysed and a group of amines found which, when administered to six migraine sufferers, brought on the well-known symptoms. In this fractional cluster of amines, a substance called betaphenylethylamine was detected and this was then focused on individually. When 3 mg of this amine – the minimum amount found in a two-ounce bar of chocolate – was given to selected subjects, an attack was precipitated. The tyramine puzzle was solved, and another piece slotted into the jigsaw. A further piece comes from the presence of another amine in some cheeses and certain alcoholic drinks – histamine, which is a powerful blood vessel dilator and which could act on the arteries producing pain and other symptoms. Other 'pressor amines' have been found, such as octopamine (in citrus fruits) and 5-hydroxytryptamine (5HT) – in tomatoes, pineapples and bananas – which is a central vasoactive substance in the biochemistry of migraine attacks. Each of these amines can work separately or in combination in a body that lacks the enzymes to rid the blood or tissues of them. It may well be also that fried and fatty foods make the intestines absorb more amines than they otherwise would, acting as a kind of lubricant to the enzyme deficiency mechanism.

Capsule given to sufferers	No effect	Headache effect
	%	%
Lactose	60	6
Tyramine	20	80

Hot dogs and ice cream

The action of these various amines on the blood vessels provides a unified biochemical picture of enzyme deficiency as a central migraine-producing mechanism. However, these are not the only chemical substances that will produce headaches and other symptoms. In recent years, with the massive spread of Chinese restaurants and take-aways, in the US, the UK and elsewhere, more monosodium glutamate has come into our diet. MSG is a white soluble substance introduced into food both as a preservative (in various frozen foods and sauces) and a flavour enhancer, and is used fairly freely in Chinese restaurant kitchens. It crops up in other forms too. For instance, in his book *More Than Two Aspirin*, Dr Seymour

Diamond, director of a migraine clinic in Chicago, ticks off some examples for a patient whose headaches seemed to be dietary in nature: 'Japanese *teriyaki*, kosher chicken soup, matza ball soup, even some everyday "normal" green pea soup.' If a tiny quantity is given to susceptible subjects MSG can cause headaches, a burning feeling in the face and a sensation of pressure on the chest. So it looks as if this particular chemical, somehow, is interfering with the body's mechanism in much the same way as certain amines, though MSG's biochemical pathways are clearly different from those of tyramine, for example.

Similarly, the preservative sodium nitrite found in frankfurters, bacon and other cured meats can induce a headache in certain people – the graphically titled 'Hot dog headache'.

Then there is the brief (lasting but a few minutes) though severe frontal head pain associated with eating ice cream. This is brought on by the cold food coming into direct contact with the lower part of the pharynx (the oropharynx) and seems to be the effect of excessive cold on the nervous and vascular regulation of susceptible head areas. Two American researchers, Raskin and Knittle, studied a group of fifty-nine migraine sufferers (thirty-seven women, twenty-two men) and found that no fewer than ninety-three per cent of them – fifty-five that is – were prone to ice cream headache, which suggests that the migraineur has to take special care. He is the one whose vasomotor regulation is most erratic and therefore most likely to show his reaction to intense cold as a vascular phenomenon.

Coping with dietary migraine: some suggestions

It is important to *know* what you are eating and drinking. This may seem self-evident but the migraineur must make sure by keeping a careful record of food intake. The memory is an unreliable source of information. Can you remember everything you ate and drank (and in what quantities) yesterday? How about the day before? Without a comprehensive record you cannot isolate the dietary factors operating in your own case and thence try to combat them. The writer Santayana said something that could have been aimed directly at migraineurs everywhere: 'Those who cannot remember the past are condemned to repeat it.'

Regulate the *timing of meals*. We know that skipped meals or slimming diets can lead to blood sugar deficiency. But whereas the non-sufferer can make good an inadequate breakfast or lunch by a compensatory snack later, the migraineur cannot. A 'chain reaction' seems to get triggered off that no amount of subsequent eating will arrest. Of course if you are an orthodox Jew or a Muslim with compulsory fast periods during Yom Kippur or the month of Ramadan your susceptibility to migraine is, literally, in the lap of the gods. On the other hand, self-willed fasting such as is dictated by a health farm regimen or strict slimming can be controlled. You may decide that the advantages of fewer migraine attacks more than offset the gain of a few pounds in weight. Incidentally, the over fifties often notice that more or less lifelong migraine begins to let up as they develop a middle-age spread. Some doctors believe that this weight gain or increase in blood sugar levels could be responsible, though this is by no means proven. So don't make a virtue of a waistline like Falstaff's!

Plan ahead your daily diet. Try finding time to sit down to a cooked meal instead of the usual sandwich for lunch, and remember to eat something mid-afternoon if for some reason (such as staggered hours) you have to take a very early midday meal. When going out in the evening, make eating something as customary as taking a bath or washing your hair. If you are going to a party then obviously alcohol consumption is the chief thing to watch. But do experiment. You may find you can drink white wine but not red or that hard liquor agrees with you more than any sorts of wines or aperitifs.

Remember too that, even if alcohol is not instrumental in your attack, the hustle and bustle of a hot, noisy room may be.

During an attack, try to eat and drink something, if only a little. The best sorts of foods are those with high carbohydrate content which you could take in the form of starch or sugar. The range of foodstuffs in these categories is enormous. The problem is really one of overcoming one's lack of inclination to eat during attacks, particularly severe ones. This is where the migraineur, like the slimmer or anyone on a special diet such as the vegetarian, is helped by developing an interest in cooking and food preparation. It is an interest that will never be under-utilised.

Try a systematic *elimination schedule*. Cut out cheese (especially the tyramine-rich matured varieties like Stilton, Brie, Emmentaler or Camembert) for as long as a month. Watch the effects and if the attacks have abated substantially (or completely) then you have found the culprit. If the attacks continue at the same rate, then go back to cheese and cut out fried food for a similar period. And so on.

Regulate the abstinence period according to the timing of your attacks. Less frequent attacks (say at several weeks intervals) will mean that you may have to forgo a certain food for as much as two months before you can assess its contribution to your migraine. Try not to cheat. Even a small amount of food, say one ounce of hot dog, can be enough to produce a headache.

If you have *children*, try to apply the same sort of monitoring system on their food intake. They are more likely to keep sugar levels up through the consumption of sweets and biscuits, but for every candy bar that may help there's a piece of chocolate or packet of potato crisps that will do the opposite.

Only a systematic examination of your diet will be of use, if only to eliminate likely precipitants. This can be difficult at times, if not impossible, when pressures at work force you to miss a meal or eat the wrong things. But keep trying. Then, in the words of Sherlock Holmes, when you have eliminated the impossible what is left must be the truth. Or very nearly.

9

Women and Children

*'I'm very brave generally,' he went on in a low voice, 'only
today I happen to have a headache.'*
Lewis Carroll, *Through the Looking Glass*

It is said that when a Parisian woman buys a two-piece swimsuit to
take with her to St Tropez, she always gets two tops, one normal size
one larger. The reason? Being a meticulous dresser with an eagle eye
for detail, she knows that the size of her breasts varies quantifiably
from week to week and, being forewarned, she prefers to be fore-
armed. Most women are less concerned over such minutiae in what
they wear, but they *are* aware of certain bodily changes, some
uncomfortable, that regularly take place. They know too that these
are intimately related to the menstrual cycle.

Hormone activity

At birth the female baby holds, in her uterus, the basis of up to
500,000 eggs which remain dormant until the age of puberty. Then,
every month, an egg is released from one of the ovaries into the
Fallopian tube, but leaves behind a small sac or follicle that grows
into an endocrine or hormone gland, the *corpus luteum*, which
produces the hormone progesterone. Progesterone acts on the uterus
to make it ready for a fertilised egg. But if one does not materialise,
the *corpus luteum* withers away, and the uterus deprived of hormone, sheds its lining – a process that causes menstrual bleeding.
Within a couple of weeks of the bleeding coming to an end the
process starts all over again. From ovulation (egg release) to menstruation is about two weeks though the cycle from there varies a
little so that the whole process can take from three to five weeks.

It is this hormonal activity that appears to be responsible for some
of the physiological and indeed emotional changes in women at cer-

tain times of the month, though it must be said that only recently have doctors began to come to grips with endocrinological phenomena and still have large gaps in their knowledge. Nevertheless it does seem irrefutable that the hormone changes that accompany menstruation are in some way linked in certain sufferers to migrainous attacks. According to the Dutch neurologist Professor G. W. Bruyn of the Utrecht Central Military Hospital: 'It is not to be expected that endocrinological factors . . . will completely explain the riddle, inasmuch as these do not appear to be operative in a third to a half of women and all the men with migraine.' However, Bruyn adds that hormones are 'a co-determinant in the migraine pattern'. Just how many women do suffer from 'menstrual migraine'? The answer to this depends on how one defines the term 'menstruation'. Of the four weeks in the monthly cycle, women regularly report to their doctors headaches in the pre-menstrual week, the week of the period itself and for a week or so *after* the period, a total of three out of four! In other words how many of these attacks are linked to the menstrual cycle itself and how many would, over this three-week span, have occurred anyway? Most experts have only a foggy idea about this though, historically, it has been an accepted medical orthodoxy that 'menstrual migraine' does exist. In 1660 Van der Linden, a Dutch physician, described the Marchioness Brandenburg's headache as a 'hemicrania *menstrua*', while Robert Whytt writing a hundred years later, stated emphatically that 'women liable to these periodic headaches suffer most severely about the menstrual periods; at which time it is well known that issues and other sores become generally more painful . . . than other parts.'

Modern research has refined these generalisations but only in recent years, with the establishment of sophisticated biochemical techniques of analysis and highly rigorous statistical methods. Nevertheless, curiosities persist. As recently as 1953 a Swedish researcher, Ask-Upmark, concluded that female migraineurs (or migraineuses) are blonde, blue-eyed, large breasted and with inverted nipples – an amazing generalisation in the eyes of doctors working in parts of the world where typical Scandinavian features, let alone inverted nipples, are less frequently met with in their migraine patients.

Menstruation
It seems that migraine is connected with endocrinological factors for four main reasons:

1. In some women migraine attacks start around the onset of menstruation, at puberty.

2. Migraine attacks and monthly periods come close together in time.

3. In some women migraine disappears during pregnancy.

4. Migraine usually disappears after the menopause or sterilisation.

Statistically speaking, there is still relatively inadequate information on any of these points. In his study of 9000 schoolchildren in Uppsala, Bo Bille found that more girls (6·4 per cent) in the thirteen to fifteen age range had migraine than in the pre-pubertal range (2·4 per cent) but, of course, this older group may by definition have been more stressed by taxing schoolwork than girls in the primary range – a suggestion supported by the fact that among *boys* the figures also rose for the higher age groups; and stress (see Chapter 10) is a frequently-cited trigger factor in migraine for people of *all* ages.

When it comes to adult women, the relationship of menstruation to migraine is just as ill-defined – although many sufferers are convinced that there is a close link. A researcher as long ago as 1912 concluded a study with the assertion that more than a third of women with migraine relate their attacks to their periods but, through the years, this study and many more recent ones have looked more and more statistically suspect. The reason for this is that mostly these researchers have relied on taking notes from the sufferers who themselves have not charted their attacks accurately enough to be useful. Much of the data has come from surveys using questionnaires, which can be notoriously unreliable. Certainly there is still a lot of disagreement over how many attacks occur regularly just before or during menstruation. Dr Katherina Dalton looked carefully at fifty-two women's attacks and found that they occurred in the pre-menstrual days and during menstruation itself in just over sixty per cent of all cases. Another piece of research, by Epstein, took as its sample 142 healthy women and found only about seventeen per cent had such a pattern of attacks! A still lower figure, of only five per cent, is arrived at for the 'true' menstrual migraine – that is headaches around the first day of bleeding. The only way one can know with any degree of certainty is for the individual sufferer to do for menstruation what she should do for food intake and *keep a chart* for at least six months so that the pattern has time to form clearly.

As well as migrainous symptoms, many women experience uncomfortable swelling of ankles and fingers and puffed eyelids, all of which are related to an excess of water being retained by the body in the form of tissue fluid. This fluid retention or oedema is interesting when associated with migraine because the two sets of symptoms may well be related. During the early part of the menstrual cycle, before ovulation and before progesterone is secreted, the body secretes another hormone, oestrogen, in the form of oestradiol. The overall level of oestradiol in the body is, at this time, unusually high, a fact which can affect the mechanism regulating fluid levels to such an extent that 'waterlogging' takes place. It may be that, in about half of all women sufferers, this oestrogen-induced water retention is related in some way to their migraines. No one yet knows for sure whether it is or not, and the evidence is slightly against concluding that the water retention actually 'causes' the migraine. This is because migraine attacks cannot be prevented by drawing off water through artificially increasing urine flow (diuresis), nor can attacks be precipitated experimentally by doctors by drug-induced fluid retention or by getting volunteers to imbibe huge quantities of water.

As oestradiol levels (and the tendency to fluid retention) increase so progesterone levels fall, and it is this delicate balance of hormones that has also been studied in itself in the search for the key to menstruation-related migraines. It is known that, in some women, relief from migraine can come from a rise in progesterone levels, whether this is administered by their doctors or whether it occurs naturally as a result of pregnancy. However, though progesterone is remarkably beneficial in some cases, it could be so, not so much for itself, as for its ability to redress the oestradiol imbalance. Certainly the mere lack of progesterone does not appear to be responsible for migraine.

Generally, the hormonal side of 'menstrual' migraine research has been an inconclusive one, with theories being constantly undermined by subsequent observations. Recently a small-scale study of menstrual migraine sufferers found no significant difference in their overall hormone levels compared to a control group even though progesterone and oestrogen levels were a bit higher. When these sufferers' attacks were looked at in detail alongside their carefully measured hormone levels, there did not seem to be any connection. The ebb and flow of hormones, their respective levels in relation to each other, were not factors in precipitating attacks. On the other hand, hormone activity is still something that medical science has a lot to find out about. Current thinking is that oestrogen may undergo local bio-chemical changes and produce effects so far undetected, but just what these changes and their effects might be will remain the subject of speculation until more systematically-gleaned evidence is forthcoming. The same is true of serotonin which, as we saw in Chapter 6, appears to be of central importance in the chain of events leading to a migraine headache. Serotonin, too, appears to be implicated in menstrual migraine, possibly as a result of oestrogen affecting blood platelet activity. Only scrupulously careful research will be able to tell whether this is so.

Meanwhile many, many women continue to relate their attacks to their periods, feeling no doubt two-way losers. For just as menstruation comes on regularly and often painfully, so do their migraine symptoms. Dr G. W. Bruyn summarised their plight thus:

> Migraine, like menstruation, can be called a curse,
> That does not need a nurse,
> Hardly ever pinches the purse,
> Seldom gets so much worse,
> As to put the patient in a hearse.

Pregnancy and the pill

In an article in the newsletter of the American National Migraine Foundation called 'Migraine: Woman's Biggest Headache', Ila Stanger points out that, in discussing migraine, 'one has to sweep aside the age-old misconception of the migraine sufferer as an elderly, highly neurotic neo-Victorian lady who takes to her bed at the first sign of something unpleasant'. True enough, especially in the light of the highly up-to-date association that many people, sufferers and doctors, have made between migraine and the use of oral contraceptives. Since oral contraceptives were introduced in the early 1960s it has become obvious that, provided the correct prescription schedule is strictly followed, this is easily the most reliable method (apart from sterilisation of either partner) of preventing pregnancies. At the same time it is a method that is not without its medical drawbacks so far as unwanted side-effects are concerned, and these have ranged from feelings of sickness or overweight to a few rare complications such as thrombosis or blood-clot formation in the vein. Another alleged effect, supported by a number of observations, is that migraine attacks can get worse or even start up in women on the pill, but once more the evidence is not conclusive.

Oral contraceptives consist of the two female hormones, oestrogen and progesterone, these being taken each day to prevent the ovaries from releasing eggs in just the same way as natural hormones prevent egg release during pregnancy. The most favoured type of pill is one with a high level of progesterone and a low dose of oestrogen and this combination has the effect of prolonging the pre-menstrual phase to several weeks instead of the normal few days. It also stimulates enzyme activity in the form of monoamine oxidase (MAO) which we know (Chapter 6) to be important in blood vessel behaviour, and the effect here is to make small arterial blood vessels swell and thicken to reach their largest just before menstruation. There does seem at first sight to be a situation in the body's reaction to hormones that could make for the familiar blood vessel dilatation that is a concomitant of migrainous headaches.

One study of 306 patients taking the pill showed that those who regularly had headaches before going on to an oral contraceptive schedule were prone to get more severe ones, though only about seven per cent of the total actually *started* to get headaches (and none of these with the typical classical or common migraine symptoms). Although headaches were the most frequent reason for patients changing from one type of pill to another – particularly to lower oestrogen levels because high oestrogen and headaches seem related – there is simply not enough hard data to state categorically that oral contraceptives bring with them the added risk of migraine. Certain types of pill do bring headaches and depression to certain hormonally sensitive women, perhaps to a larger degree than many people appreciate. But, so far as migraine is concerned, it is impossible to be conclusive about the pill's effects. One survey actually found a *decrease* in migraine symptoms in some women starting on oral contraception. Many women take oral contraceptives for years without any apparent effects, even though in the process the chemistry of their body has been subjected to numerous changes and fluctuations, while others react badly immediately. All one can say is that these reactions involve disturbances in their hormonal balance, abnormal enzyme and amine activity and the possibility of blood vessel changes, so it would not be surprising if migraine attacks somehow were a concomitant feature. At the Radcliffe Infirmary in Oxford, Judith Hockaday studied the relationship between migraine attacks, the menstrual cycle and hormone activity, and came to the same conclusion which she frames in a 'better safe than sorry' form: 'While it is not proven that migraine is an added risk factor, there is sufficient doubt to justify the recommendation to avoid oral contraceptives (OCC) in women with classical or complicated migraine, and in women whose vascular headaches are made worse by OCC.' This is good sense though, as is often the case, individual women have to do their own risk–benefit analysis of their particular situation. Are the pill's advantages swamped by the pain (or potential pain) of migrainous headaches? Or would an unwanted child represent an even bigger headache?

So far as pregnancy is concerned there is less disagreement among experts as to the effect on migraine attacks. Attacks unequivocally are relieved in about sixty-five to seventy-five per cent of cases, presumably as the result of major hormonal changes, almost as if nature were lightening one burden on the expectant mother. This relief is particularly marked in those women who previously had associated menstrual periods in particular with their attacks. When pregnancy is over, however, migraine returns to plague the sufferer and continues on through to the menopause, after which there is usually an improvement.

Children and migraine

When a young child complains to its mother of a headache or an upset stomach, a number of causes spring to mind, many of which are related to the everyday, energetic and adventurous nature of the complainant's activities, be this playing games or eating underripe apples. Rarely do adults think in terms of a child's headache as being migrainous, preferring quite rightly in most cases to look for factors like hyperactivity or emotional stress as the likely causes. Even doctors are often slow to diagnose migraine in children. A well-known textbook of children's diseases calls migraine 'a disease of adults' and gives it no further consideration. But this is wrong. Children *do* have migraine. Studies of patients at the Princess Margaret Migraine Clinic showed that more than half of the 2000 sufferers questioned started attacks before the age of twenty and eighteen per cent of the total before the age of ten. A large-scale study in Sweden produced an even more startling statistic: that one child in twenty-five at school is a migraineur.

Children's attacks occur more frequently than those of adults, though they are of shorter duration. Headaches often affect both sides of the head, later in life becoming one-sided, and are usually not very severe. Often abdominal pains, vomiting and visual disturbances occur, sometimes giddiness and feverishness. If these mimic the fully-blown adult migraine in terms of length of attack and frequency of occurrence, and no physical causes can be pinned down, then the child is likely to have classical or common migraine in adult life. This is particularly true of 'periodic' or 'cyclical' vomiting and it can be so for some, though by no means all, persistent cases of car or travel sickness.

For the parent or doctor it is not always easy to know just what symptoms the child really has. Parents of the children who go on to develop into adult migraine sufferers notice periods when they seemed unduly tired or listless, lacking initiative, though these mood changes are not the only more subtle ones that occur. Although there is very little evidence of visual disturbances such as the adult aura symptoms in migrainous children, they do get 'peculiar' feelings that they can scarcely articulate let alone explain. Over half these sufferers, fortunately, are rid of attacks in later years though the child whose attacks started very young, and persisted frequently, is less likely to. Around puberty the childhood version, often inseparable from a whole host of other conditions, comes of age and a genuine migraine case becomes easier to identify. At this stage, as with adults, a chart based on the Trigger Checklist is an invaluable tool to help isolate the factors at play in particular instances. One word of warning though; in monitoring your child's attacks, food intake, activities, stress times and so on, use some discretion over the degree of importance you appear to attach to the whole business. You need his or her co-operation but not at the expense of heightening fears of future attacks. Try not to 'exchange one nuisance for another'.

Treating migraine in children can never, while the causes of the condition remain unclear, be entirely satisfactory. It has to be directed towards coping with acute attacks and, if possible, preventing others from occurring.

In an acute attack, the strategy to employ is similar to that employed for adults. Get the child to a quiet darkened room and, if he or she is not vomiting, provide glucose drinks to sip. Let your child's teacher or headteacher know that attacks of this kind can occur so that similar conditions can be asked for and obtained in schooltime if necessary.

Soluble aspirin following your doctor's recommended dosage will often help, taken at four-hourly intervals, and again this should be available at school. Under these conditions a child will often fall asleep, waking up feeling better, though if sickness and vomiting are a problem then a tablet (or syrop) of metoclopramide can also be given ten minutes before the aspirin or paracetamol. Other drugs such as ergotamine tartrate that may have unwelcome side-effects are inappropriate for children, though some doctors may still try ergotamine if the measures described above seem to be failing and the child is still greatly distressed.

If migraine headaches are frequently severe and obviously having adverse effects on the child's everyday activities, it is possible to try preventive treatment. It has been found that diazepam (Valium) and chlordiazepoxide (Librium) can work well in about fifty per cent of cases and these have the advantage of few side-effects. Other prophylactic treatments include a peppermint-flavoured tablet of phenytoin and pizotifen, though there are certain drawbacks to the use of both these drugs at present.

Between about the ages of nine and fourteen some children will complain of severe and persistent headaches that are not migrainous but 'psychological' in that they result from an emotional circumstance sometimes of the parent's own making. Dr Marcia Wilkinson describes these thus: '. . . they [the headaches] may be being used either by the mother or the child to manipulate the situation . . . and often it is the mother who is being over-protective to her growing child'. The psychological explanation may turn out to be the correct one but should not be seized on too quickly. Keep it at the back of your mind until you have good reason to bring it to the front.

10

Migraine-minded: the Psychological Element

'Nothing is either good or bad but thinking makes it so.'
Shakespeare, *Hamlet*

Advances in our understanding of medicine have uncovered a paradox. As we refine our knowledge and edge step by step towards enlightenment, as we strike out and penetrate the depths of specialised lines of enquiry, we run the risk of losing sight of the whole problem by exploring its every part. Ever since the earliest times when some members of society differentiated themselves by acting as the agents of care and cure by becoming doctors to their fellow men, one principle has remained unshakeable: that to treat a person's illness you have to treat the whole person. Without the co-operation of the patient, much of what the doctor does can be diluted, if not totally wasted. The will to get well, as any doctor will acknowledge, is indispensable to the total recovery process, because surgery and pill-taking of themselves are rarely enough. Likewise, the process of *becoming* ill often has a non-physical component, a psychological or emotional strand that is inextricably, often mysteriously, enmeshed in the malfunctioning of an organ or some other bodily activity. To know what is wrong, a doctor has to explore *how* the illness arose, a skill that requires imagination and persistence on his part and a good deal of understanding.

The paradox then lies in the fact that the trend is irreversibly towards specialisation in medicine while the need for a generalised approach to illness is as strong, if not stronger, now than it was when Hippocrates was examining his patients. In their book on psychology and medicine, Jack Rachman and Clare Philips of London's Institute of Psychiatry report on their investigation of this need. They found that, although today's patient risks becoming depersonalised by the bureaucracy of hospital administration, the medical world is alert to the danger by showing itself 'more and more convinced that the consideration of the patient as an individual is at least as important as other factors in the treatment of his disease; our increasing know-ledge of psychosomatic disorders has added impetus to the demand that we should treat the patient not the disease'. These are poten-tially comforting words for any of us likely to come into first-hand contact with doctors and hospitals, and especially so if the reason for this contact is that one's problem is migraine. They are, moreover, not only a reflection of what is happening in Britain. In America Dr Seymour Diamond stated nearly ten years ago that 'The social and psychological needs of the patient should be given as much consider-ation as his physiochemical and bacteriological derangement.'

What this means, so far as migraine sufferers are concerned, is that attacks may be regarded as the ultimate physical manifestation of a series of causal links, strung together in some degree by an individual's peculiar vulnerability. This vulnerability in turn has itself a number of causes but its overall effect is to act as a pointer to a person's susceptibility to certain personal or social pressures. Unfortunately, as is so often true of migraine, this susceptibility has frequently been alluded to and often described but rarely with much regard for scientific objectivity. Is there indeed such a thing as a 'migraine personality' and if so what is it? How does this produce the responses that somehow facilitate the neuro-vascular or hormonal disruptions we know to be linked to attacks? Are migraineurs in any way 'mentally ill'? These are the psychological problems that doctors are beginning to grapple with in a more systematic way than they did in the past. Let's see what sort of conclusions they are reaching.

Migraine personality – myth or not?
Although migraine has been a battleground for many conflicting ideas and beliefs, there has, comparatively, been a large measure of agreement among experts on the so-called distinctive 'personality characteristics' of sufferers. The manner in which we react to stimuli, the personal characteristics that are responsible for stamping our actions constitute our 'personality' – a quality that psychologists spend a great deal of time in studying, measuring and describing. These characteristics are many; sociability; ruthlessness; efficiency; slovenliness and so on and so forth, and not all so-called 'personality' descriptions are particularly scientific. They are not a measure of

specific, well-defined traits but an agglomeration of personal impressions, gleaned sometimes in artificial or misleading circumstances. Take the idea of 'proud'. What does this mean? That a person is arrogant and haughty? Fussy about the people he or she is seen with? Unprepared to admit weakness? It can mean any or all of these, or even something else, according to what your viewpoint of the 'proud' person is in the first place (i.e. as his doctor, employee, spouse or enemy).

For migraineurs a number of personality profiles have been offered, many with a common core of features: Arnold Friedman, the American neurologist, describes the sufferer as one who exhibits 'adult perfectionism, rigidity, resentment, ambitiousness, efficiency, a constitutional predisposition to sustained emotional states ... inflexibility, over-conscientiousness, meticulousness, perfectionism'. This list of traits chimes with the observations of other workers in the field who, taking migraine patients as a whole, have seen in them an unusual level of perfectionism and ambition. They are, it seems, people who like to be in control of the situation and themselves, and, conversely, dislike unpredictability, indecision and uncertain events. They find it relatively difficult to relax and unwind, and to lower standards. According to one research team, migraineurs have difficulty in handling repressed feelings of hostility or anger, even that 'unresolved dependency needs and psychosexual conflicts are also frequently present'. According to one clinician, Sacks, there is a category of 'aggressive migraine' that strikes people whose emotional background is one of 'intense, chronic, repressed rage and hostility, and the function of the migraine is to provide some expression of what cannot be expressed, or even acknowledged, directly'. Sacks also identifies cases of migraine patients who are 'deeply masochistic, spiteful, chronically depressed, covertly paranoid, and sometimes overtly self-destructive'. The 'migraine personality' in these descriptions appears to be a slightly unsympathetic one, with a strong neurotic strain to it. The question is: what evidence is there that these unappealing *impressions* of psychological traits are anything more than impressions? Then there is the other side of the coin, the personality profile of the migraine sufferer that puts him in a more positive light. The British general practitioner, Dr K. M. Hay, who has made extensive studies of migraine, points out that: 'The disorder is common in artistic, literary and academic circles. It is found among people percipient and imaginative who have strong drives to communicate their ideas, or to translate them into action.' They are important people in society, scholars, musicians, company directors and so on – according to this set of impressions. What one person might see as restless inflexibility becomes for someone else a commendable striving for accuracy and a job well done. The migraine personality like the actor's masks, or *personae* from which the word is derived, can have simultaneously a sunny or a cloudy aspect. Yet the issue still remains as to whether these traits – however interpreted – really are there in the first place. We saw in Chapter 4 that until comparatively recently doctors may have held certain misconceptions about the social class of their migraine patients simply because those lower down the social scale would be less likely to consult them for the condition. Does the same sort of misconception prevail about the *personality* of sufferers?

The problem is that until very recently the group of scientists most able to offer an objective assessment, the psychologists and psychophysiologists, have virtually ignored it. Because of this, non-psychological researchers have tended to rely on the sorts of psychoanalytical or subjective impressions recorded above, and so perhaps swallow and thereafter perpetrate a mythological notion of what kind of person the migraine sufferer is. Very recently, however, psychologists have been entering into the picture and offering some challenging evidence. At the Maudsley Institute of Psychiatry, psychologist Clare Philips tried to discover how many objective studies there had been of the personality of unselected headache cases, and found only one. In assessing the 'personality' of migraine sufferers or any other group of people, it is important to ensure that the sample chosen is not biased in any way and that measures of various traits are done alongside control groups for comparison. As far as migraine patients are concerned, it is known that less than fifty per cent of headache sufferers complain to their doctors and that only a very small percentage of these go on to a specialist neurological clinic. By the time they reach their doctors the migraine sufferers have already sorted themselves out into complainers and non-complainers. Psychological research shows that 'high complainers' (about anything) tend to be more neurotic and extraverted than 'low complainers', and that the more neurotic and extraverted people are the less they appear to tolerate pain. Clinical impressions by doctors of the migraine sufferers consulting them are thus bound to be somewhat biased in favour of the personality myths. Yet, using one test based on a

Personality Questionnaire measuring neuroticism, extraversion and other traits, Philips found *no* significant differences between migraine patients and control groups. 'There was,' she affirms, 'no evidence of the oft-quoted neuroticism of this group.' This kind of objective research, she considers, will, bit by bit, smash most of the traditional beliefs about the relationship of personality to headache. Few doctors, one imagines, will persist in labelling patients in this way.

At the same time one should not forget that doctors must continue to see, in their migraine patients, some evidence of these traits, not so much as fixed personality characteristics (many of which were there perhaps from birth) but as a *response to circumstances* of severe pain and a disrupted way of life, work and leisure. When these circumstances persist over many years, is it to be wondered at that migraine sufferers appear resentful, irritable and often depressed? What the migraine sufferer is showing is an acute sensitivity or reactivity to stress situations, and that is the nature of his neuroticism.

Arousal, stress, tension and anxiety

Although, as we have seen, the idea of migraine as being closely linked to a set of personality features is one that is being critically re-examined in such a way as to threaten long-held notions, one should not undervalue the psychological component of attacks. There is no doubt that, whatever else they may or may not be, migraine sufferers are distinctly sensitive to certain kinds of situations which act as triggers to their symptoms. Sensitivity to arousing or stressful situations is, in some degree, common to us all. When we hear an unusual bump downstairs in the dead of night or watch the home team score the winning goal, our bodies automatically react in a combination of different ways – pulse and heart rates step up, breathing varies, stomach muscles contract, perspiration or saliva flow and so on. These measurable physiological responses are the body's 'red alert' system for meeting and coping with the situation, whether it be frightening, difficult or just stirringly pleasurable. We all have them, though not necessarily to the same degree for a given situation. What worries you greatly may leave your best friend unmoved and vice versa.

With migraine, the sufferer is highly reactive or 'emotionally labile', having a body that responds to stress situations (or those about to happen) in an extreme way. Seymour Diamond asserts that: 'Headache patients as a whole tend to build in themselves lives with too many environmental demands. They are extremely sensitive to this overload. They suffer situational anxieties . . . Stress situations of life, such as menopause, puberty, changes of school, changes of job, paralyse their adapting mechanism.' Some of the people who react unfavourably in this way may not necessarily be migraine sufferers, but may instead have the so-called tension-headaches, which are mostly bilateral and caused by muscular contraction at key pain-producing points in the region of the head, neck and shoulders. Some may be migraineurs *and* tension headache sufferers, while others migraine sufferers solely.

The tension headache sufferer's main problem is the failure to relax, so treatment usually consists of some kind of relaxation exercise allied with drug therapy. But for this kind of headache, as for migraine (which has a greater range of symptoms), it clearly helps if one can avoid stressful situations in the first place. It is not uncommon for tension headaches to plague people who, in addition to doing an exacting job, fill their 'free' time with equally strenuous activities like being secretary of numerous clubs, sitting on committees and taking a tireless part in all sorts of sports and similar recreations. On holiday, after a few days adjusting to the slower pace, the tension headache may disappear.

Migraine sufferers also sometimes find it hard to relax, to sit back and let things just happen: they tend to get anxious and remain so even when they might be 'enjoying themselves'. However, it is not simply anxiety that contributes to their attacks. In the course of his long experience of migraine Dr K. M. Hay came across one patient who worked in the tote office of a travelling race course because she was so taken with the excitement of the racing world. She did frenzied odds calculations at high speed while the races were being run and this she also found a thrill. Next day, without fail, she got her migraine attacks. The excess of emotional arousal, it seemed, had not been filtered off overnight and had somehow carried over to activate a painful physiological response. The Professor of Medicine at Cambridge University, Ivor Mills, recently gave a lecture on 'Migraine and Man's Environment', in which he discussed the arousal mechanism in relation to stress-induced migraine. He pointed out that attacks may occur while the arousal is at its peak or just after the peak, a let-up phenomenon whereby decreased work load seems to bring 'weekend migraine'. This could come about because high arousal engenders an 'underlying depression' which stays dormant until the let-up period. Then it comes to the surface, with associated migraine attacks. Depression and migraine are often seen together in patients; perhaps nearly half of all headaches are associated with chronic recurrent depression accompanied by sleep disturbance.

Various anxiety-making or high-arousal conditions can be related to migraine, making it in part a 'psychosomatic' condition. How big a part psychology plays is a highly debatable point. Many migraine sufferers are by no means neurotic or emotionally unstable, and even those who are can have attacks precipitated by situations that should not have such effects, such as pleasant experiences or prolonged and unbroken sleep. In many respects it is all too easy to point to a restless or thrusting type of person and see the ideal breeding ground for attacks which, by their often bizarre nature, seem to have a strong 'psychological' component. On the other hand, there are too many grey areas in our understanding of the psychosomatic element in illness as a whole for any observation to be conclusive. The best one can do at present is look to psychological and emotional factors as contributing to the triggering mechanism.

Psychology and treatment – new horizons?

One way of gauging the part played by psychosomatic factors in bringing on attacks is to see what effects are produced on headaches and other symptoms by psychotherapeutic techniques. At their briefest these techniques are, in the view of one researcher, a short catalogue of advice to sufferers. Something along the following lines:

> The world is not perfect so don't try to reach perfection
> Don't be a slave to the clock
> You can't please everyone
> Be less critical of yourself
> . . . . . . and so on . . . . . .

If you are a sufferer and find that this kind of do-it-yourself psychotherapy actually works, then well and good. If it does not, perhaps some other psychological treatment – dealt with in detail in a later chapter – may be more appropriate, be this relaxation therapy, hypnosis, biofeedback or tranquillisers. One Dutch professor of psychiatry specialising in psychosomatic disorders claims a certain level of success by using combined psychotherapeutic techniques, both 'talking treatments' and drug regimens, but there are still relatively few doctors willing or able to practise these 'multimedia' methods. For the most part, treatments for migraine of a psychological kind are like any others, in that they may be tried out individually and continued with if they seem to work. So far as the patient is concerned, he or she must not be surprised if neurologists scorn the idea of some kind of partial psychological explanation for attacks, usually preferring to think purely in terms of readjusting the neuro-vascular mechanisms to put things right. Nor, on the contrary, should it seem odd if your doctor asks you what appear to be very peripheral questions about your emotional state before attacks, your general relationship with others or your hopes and fears. Neither side is wholly right or wholly wrong. Certain situations can build up a psychological overload in some people which has a physical outcome, but, on the other hand, even extreme stress, like the appalling conditions in a concentration camp, will not necessarily precipitate migraine attacks. There are simply no common personality or situational factors that can be pinned down, even though they seem to remain, naggingly, in the wings of the migraine scenario, as one of the currents that support what has been called 'the flight into illness'.

11

Doctors and Treatments

*'Medicine is the art of pouring drugs of which one knows
nothing into a patient of which one knows even less.'*

Voltaire

The curious, often vivid nature of migraine attacks, especially as
manifested in their 'classical' forms, has over many centuries generated an equally graphic range of alleged treatments, including
magic. In the Middle Ages doctors worked their way through all the
drugs, potions and mixtures known to medical practice and, when
these failed, resorted to favoured standbys such as blood letting. By
the early 1800s the physician and writer Heberden conceded that
bleeding was 'detrimental' but still persisted in trying to cure
patients with a catalogue of concoctions that included Peruvian bark,
camphor, sneezing powders, hemlock and opium, not to mention
such measures as 'opening the temporal artery, and drawing of some
teeth'. He claimed most success with 'blisters behind the ears' that
appeared to temper the violence of attacks and, when all else failed, a
'lasting cure' based on tartar and a lot of opium, taken at bedtime for
six nights in a row. A lasting cure indeed! Other remedies have
included nitroglycerine tablets, Indian hemp and repeated stimulation of the sympathetic nervous system, while during the American
Civil War General Ulysses Grant reckoned that his chronic migraine
headache was instantly cured by his receiving word that General Lee
wanted to surrender his armies! Doctors have in the past experimented ingeniously with all kinds of methods of treatment, from
drastic skull surgery to fanciful but mild medicines, and sufferers
have reported a variety of personal experiences of cures and attempted cures. All this activity failed to produce a definitive solution
and, in our own time, more scientifically-based therapies have likewise not proved to be the all-purpose answer. The wonder drug has

not been discovered. Yet this does not stop many doctors (and, understandably, sufferers) from hoping – expecting even – that it will be found, even though on balance it seems unlikely that this will ever be the case.

Migraine is a multi-factorial illness in a number of different ways; it involves a number of features of the body's neuro-vascular equipment; it is triggered off by one or a number of different precipitants; it plagues people with a very wide range of symptoms. In short, the more scientists study it the more complicated in terms of interlocking pieces does the puzzle appear. Over and above all this there is the human element, the individual's particular reactivity to causal situations, external influence, bodily rhythms and cycles and, most important, to courses of treatment. So many variables in the equation must make it impossible to think of a 'cure' for migraine in the same way as we regard antibiotics as the cure for certain infections, or surgical operations as the remedy for other types of physical malfunctioning. Migraine has to be thought of in the same terms as various other conditions such as epilepsy, in that doctors already have a range of drugs at their disposal for dealing with certain aspects, such as pain killers, substances for influencing blood vessel responses, drugs to modify blood characteristics or neurological behaviour – and from these they have a choice which, by trial and error, may lead to improvements in specific relevant body mechanisms. In addition there are non-pharmacological treatment measures, again aimed to specific targets. The fact that no one measure can be held up as *the* cure or treatment is not necessarily a reason for gloom, neither is the fact that such an all-purpose measure is unlikely to be discovered. Migraine sufferers can, with the help of their doctors and some sensible management of their lives, find a good deal of hope and relief, perhaps more than they realise. Better by far to be optimistic about the efficacy of the tools that are to hand, than suffer the added despondency of grasping at one of the most elusive of medical straws.

Treatments available (if you want them)

A forty-year-old woman walks into her doctor's consulting room and complains of a series of symptoms which he quickly diagnoses as migraine. As the doctor goes on to uncover more details that may help him to treat his patient, he will certainly ask how long the attacks have been going on and will not be surprised to learn that they started at least ten years previously. So why did his patient choose to come only now? Are the headaches getting unbearable whereas in the past they could be coped with? Has the patient recently done something that could have had a profound effect such as taking to using oral contraceptives? Is she at the start of a crash slimming course? Somewhere along the line the doctor may uncover some important factors which he can bear in mind in prescribing courses of treatment. At the same time he will be struck once more by the fact that many sufferers endure their attacks for many years – half of them never coming to him for help – unaware perhaps of what can be done, sometimes perhaps even a little ashamed to bother their physician. But there *are* things that can be done and they *should* consult him.

In the absence of a cure that will free a sufferer from migraine for all time, treatments available fall into two main categories:

1. Preventative, which involves both drug therapy as well as trying to establish and maintain an environment that is not conducive to attacks. In this category come the 'attack abortion' treatments for nipping in the bud an imminent attack before it has a chance to flower.

2. Symptomatic, which involves treating the pain and discomforts of attacks, both mild and chronic, in order to bring a measure of relief. They range from the widely used analgesic or pain killer, aspirin, to tranquillising drugs like Valium to induce sleep. So far there is no drug or other treatment for halting a fully-developed attack.

Symptomatic treatments
When Arnold Friedman carried out his classic study of 5000 headache sufferers and the many different drugs tried on them, he concluded that only a very few drugs were effective. At the same time it is generally accepted that, when an attack is under way, one can make things better by some very simple measures: find a dark, quiet room to rest in undistracted; avoid lying out flat, but keep the head raised, sip iced water containing glucose if you are not feeling too sick (and if you are, make sure you restore the sugar level in the blood by taking glucose as soon as possible afterwards either in water or separately); try applying a slight pressure to the temporal artery on the painful side: it can be felt quite distinctly at a point about two inches forward from the top of the ear. Measures such as these, in many cases, bring partial relief, though it is recorded that some people take

quite the opposite measures: they play violent sports, get angry and even – back to the eighteenth century – take sneezing powder. All these fairly explosive activities have appeared to alleviate matters. There is no permanent harm done in experimenting with them, though you may prefer to bear with a migraine attack than deliberately start a slanging match with the person nearest to you in order to try to assuage it.

Pain killers

As well as seeking out the right kind of environment, it is of course important to try to mitigate the pain, and by far the most readily available analgesic is *aspirin* which probably helps more people than any other pharmacological preparation. Aspirin (acetylsalicylic acid) belongs to the family of drugs known as the 'salicylates', developed from salicylic acid which was first discovered in the nineteenth century in Germany. It is one of the most widely used drugs, often for the wrong reasons: for example, many people pop a couple of tablets in their mouth in the vague belief that they will 'calm the nerves' and lift depression; others consider them a good preparation to induce sleep. In fact, the prime effect of aspirin is to relieve pain, in the same way that, in earlier periods, narcotics such as opium were employed. Unlike opium or alcohol, however, aspirin does not stupefy the person who takes it nor does it lead, after long-term use, to tolerance or physical dependence. Its action is not such as to work specifically on toothache or headache or painful muscles but to generally dull one's conscious awareness of pain, by acting on that part of the brain that translates nerve impulses from troublesome areas of the body into feeling.

At the same time aspirin has various other effects. It will bring down the migraineur's temperature (antipyretic); reduce any inflammation and, according to recent research, reduce the level of prostaglandins which are thought to be implicated in the migraine process. On the other hand, taken in high doses, aspirin has other, less beneficial effects of particular interest to migraine sufferers, such as lowering of blood sugar content, increasing fluid retention and stepping up the body's metabolic or energy-using rate. If taken in overdose quantities, aspirin can even cause migraine-like symptoms such as deafness, noises in the ears, nausea and a dull headache – a condition called 'salicylism'.

Another effect of very large doses is on the digestive system – causing gastro-intestinal upset and sometimes bleeding which cumulatively may lead to anaemia. Aspirin is also dangerous when used too freely for people with specific problems such as heart disease or impaired function of kidneys, liver or blood.

If taken properly, that is according to your doctor's advice, aspirin can be a valuable front-line aid, at its most effective if taken and absorbed before the stomach becomes inactive early on in a migraine attack. Generally the more severe the headache the less easily the body absorbs the aspirin, a phenomenon studied at the Princess Margaret Clinic by Glyn Volans and attributed to gastro-intestinal 'stasis' probably as a result of heightened activity of the sympathetic nervous system. To aid absorption the drug metoclopramide may be given by doctors to stimulate normal stomach activity, alongside the easily assimilable aspirin in soluble or effervescent form. Soluble or effervescent aspirin also helps to reduce gastro-intestinal upsets (sickness) which are further alleviated if the aspirin is taken after food and drink. The use of the anti-emetic (or anti-vomiting) drug metoclopramide is now fairly well established, because like other anti-emetics it acts directly to reduce dopamine levels which are probably implicated in causing migraine, and has the added bonus of helping the body to absorb aspirin normally given in tablet form about ten minutes afterwards.

Some people have a natural, implacable allergy to aspirin, in which case another analgesic *paracetamol* may be used. Like aspirin the dosages recommended by doctors are usually around four times daily and, like aspirin, paracetamol lowers body temperature. It has no anti-inflammation properties. Excessive doses of paracetamol have, of course, their dangers; not in affecting, as does aspirin, the gastro-intestinal tract and causing bleeding but rather in damaging the liver and kidneys. So although the stomach upsets do not occur, use paracetamol according to prescription, and remember that it is available in effervescent form. Metoclopramide to stimulate normal stomach contractions and prevent vomiting is also used in tandem with paracetamol. Until fairly recently *phenacetin* was also frequently used as a pain reliever but, if your doctor formerly prescribed it and does so no longer, it is because the side-effects of the drug (in causing kidney damage) are, in certain countries, including Britain, reckoned to be too dangerous.

Many proprietary brands of analgesics contain both paracetamol and aspirin as well as other pain killers such as *codein* phosphate. For several hundred years the stimulant *caffeine* has found some favour as a treatment, though strictly speaking its usefulness in migraine therapy is limited to the way it can help the body to assimilate ergotamine tartrate (see below). Caffeine is found in various easily available forms, notably tea and coffee, and in many a chemist's-shop 'pick-me-up' and pain reliever, though its stimulant effects are often not in accord with the migraine sufferer's desire for rest and quiet.

The ergotamine story

Of all the symptomatic treatments for migraine, one drug has for years now stood out from the rest as the most effective measure to combat the severe throbbing headache, as opposed to the vague aches that often precede it, and which can sometimes be relieved by aspirin or another analgesic. That substance is *ergotamine tartrate* (often simply 'ergotamine'), a powerful preparation isolated from ergot and, in fact, a derivative of another powerful drug LSD (lysergic acid). Ergot derives in turn from a fungus, *Claviceps purpura*, which can flourish in the dampness of badly-made granaries. In its raw state it is not a medicine but a poison. During periods of war or famine when people have been obliged to eat what was to hand, including mouldy grain supplies, the fungus produced 'ergotism' – a severe illness causing its victims burning pains and even the loss of limbs through gangrene. The modern pharmaceutical preparation is still potentially harmful, despite its value in dealing with about eighty per cent of acute migraine cases. It has always been absolutely forbidden as a migraine treatment for women during pregnancy and for people with various diseases of the liver and kidneys.

Ergotamine is not used as a matter of course initially but, once decided upon by doctors, is given as early as possible for an acute attack. It is not known precisely how it operates on the body but it is certainly a strong vasoactive drug. It constricts the small blood vessels and perhaps puts into reverse the trend towards dilatation (see Chapter 5) of cranial arteries that is thought to play a crucial role in the stabbing pulsations of migrainous headaches. Ergotamine exists in various forms: as tablets (e.g. Migril, Cafergot, Femergin, Orgraine, Ergodryl capsules); suppositories (Cafergot); inhalers (Medihaler-ergotamine) and injections. Other proprietary names include Lingraine and Bellergal. For all these, best results are obtained if ergotamine is given early and in the most appropriate form, and here the sufferer must be advised by his or her doctor. A person may like to take tablets but, if these are absorbed very slowly, another method has to be tried. In other cases persistent vomiting may mean that suppositories are the most efficacious method of administering the drug. Although effective, ergotamine is not without its attendant dangers of side-effects. It is also not an all-purpose drug. It will treat symptoms but will not prevent them from starting up and should never be taken prophylactically in the vain hope that it will. The drug is hardly ever used with children.

The problem with ergotamine is that, as work at specialist migraine clinics over the past few years has revealed, an effective dose is only a little less than a dose that produces side-effects, the most common of which are nausea, vomiting, headache, diarrhoea and a general feeling of being unwell. In other words, the recommended maximum dose per week is 10–12 mg (say six Migril tablets, six Cafergot suppositories or twelve Cafergot tablets) but many sufferers exceed this because they persist for hours with repeated doses of the drug for a splitting headache whereas ergotamine will, if it is to work at all, usually bring relief within an hour. Having taken an overdose, a sufferer will get the side-effect symptoms described above which, of course, resemble migraine. So they take even more ergotamine to get rid of it in one vicious and habit-forming circle. These dangers of self-poisoning are so real (affecting perhaps as many as eight per cent of headache sufferers taking the drug) that ergotamine after a long innings seems to be on its way out. Perhaps its death blow was dealt by the medical directors of two London Migraine clinics who encapsulated their extensive experience of working with ergotamine in a letter, headed 'Ergotamine tartrate overdose', to the *British Medical Journal*. They wrote:

Sir, At the Charing Cross Hospital Migraine Clinic and the Princess Margaret Migraine Clinic we have seen a number of patients who, in our opinion, are suffering from ergotamine tartrate overdose. These can be divided into two groups: those who habitually take one or more milligrams a day and who suffer daily headaches and nausea, the characteristic of the headache being that it is relieved only by further doses of ergotamine; and a very much smaller group who have signs of ergotism. In our experience ergotamine headache may occur with doses as little as one milligram daily of ergotamine tartrate by mouth or 0·25 mg daily by intra-muscular injection. Our work at the Charing Cross Hospital and Princess Margaret Clinic has led us to think that an anti-emetic such as 10 mg of metoclopramide followed fifteen minutes later by an effervescent preparation of aspirin or paracetamol is the best treatment for most acute attacks of migraine.

F. Clifford Rose

Migraine Clinic
Charing Cross Hospital
London W6

Marcia Wilkinson

Princess Margaret Migraine Clinic
London EC1

This unequivocal conclusion has been getting support from other sources. Some neurologists at the University of Oulu in Finland studied 600 migraine patients they had personally attended over five years and found that forty-three of them had taken more than 10 mg of ergotamine, i.e. an excessive amount, for at least six months, and nearly half these had signs of ergot poisoning. The most serious consequence of overdosage they found was vascular complications. So the message is clear: ergotamine is effective but dangerous if not handled with the utmost care by doctor and patient. It is imperative, if you are a regular user of the drug or are likely to become one, to know precisely how much you are taking regularly, bearing in mind that some preparations, e.g. Migril or Cafergot suppositories, contain twice as much as others.

And remember, ergotamine is specifically useful for migraine, so much so in fact that some doctors have even defined migraine as a condition that responds to the drug. This definition may be faulty but the premise on which it is built is not. Ergotamine if used at all is for migrainous headaches, and *for no other kinds*.

Treating pain trigger areas

Between attacks, migraine sufferers usually have no abnormal physical symptoms, except perhaps for the presence of small sensitive areas in the muscles of the scalp and shoulder girdle.

Some sufferers are rarely free from some soreness in the head and often get twinges of pain when particular spots on the scalp are touched by their hairdresser. These spots may be as small as half a centimetre across but doctors can identify them fairly easily, either by slight pressure (getting a reaction from his patient) or by the subtle changes in the 'feel' and texture of the skin and scalp tissue at the critical points. It is fairly commonplace for some doctors to inject a mixture of lignocaine, which is a local anaesthetic, and a tiny

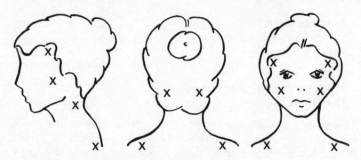

Common pain trigger areas in migraine

amount of adrenaline into up to four of these spots and the surrounding areas. Initially there is a sharp pain because the spots are so hypersensitive, but relief is quick and often visual symptoms of migraine are cleared up as well as the headache. The relief achieved by these local anaesthetics appears to last on average about three weeks, certainly far longer than the effects of the lignocaine itself. One advantage of trigger area injections is that ergotamine treatment is avoided, though why they should be so effective is not certain. In Britain most of the cases so far have been patients at the Birmingham Migraine Clinic where over a hundred sufferers have been treated in this way, and the results have been encouraging. Only time and the experiences of other sufferers having these injections will decide whether they become a regular feature of the battery of symptomatic, distress-relieving measures currently being used.

12

More About Treatment: Prevention Possibilities

'Oh! that the Healer's art and skill
Could dissipate this pain, this ill!'
Anon.

At its most effective, good medical care is essentially two-sided, involving both doctor and patient in a reciprocal relationship, and nowhere is this better illustrated than in the management of migraine. In the last chapter we saw how certain therapeutic measures could be taken to relieve attacks once they had got under way and how the sufferer needs to be aware of what drugs he is taking, for what reasons and in what quantities. Similarly, on the other side of treatment – prevention – the migraineur can play a part, and an even more important one, in contributing to his own welfare. Preventive measures start with the sufferer and with his unique knowledge of himself, his life style and his likes, dislikes, reactions and outlook.

In Chapter 7 we looked at the various trigger factors that can precipitate attacks. This is the place to start, by avoiding the circumstances and situations that you know to be potentially aggravating or that you suspect could be to blame. If, as has been suggested, migraine is precipitated roughly fifty per cent of the time by 'psychogenic' factors, namely tense or anxious states of mind occasioned by stress, fatigue, insomnia and depression, then a careful look at one's own emotional cycle could be worthwhile. Ideally (and this is only an ideal state of affairs) one is aiming at avoiding emotional peaks and troughs, because high levels of stimulation and excitement as well as gloomy phases are conducive to migraine in those susceptible to attack.

This ideal of balance and calm in one's emotional life is to be sought after in other ways; 'moderation in all things' being the rule. This means avoiding too much over-rich food or too much of any substance that could act unfavourably, including alcohol; keeping the body in good physical shape with regular exercise, like walking or swimming, but avoiding over-exertion; trying to steer clear of extremes of heat, light and noise which may necessitate a quiet lunch on a park bench instead of the more congenial atmosphere of the canteen. In many respects the sort of approach to diet, exercise and health specifically needed by the migraine sufferer to avoid attacks is identical to what everyone in the population should be aiming for. In dealing with the subject of prevention of attacks, a compendious home medical guide published in America a few years back, offered the following advice: '. . . an effort should be made to improve general health and nutrition. Any obvious mental strain or anxiety should if possible be corrected, and the patient should avoid becoming overtired.' Good advice for anyone and everyone whether they suffer from persistent headaches or not.

Preventive treatments

If a migraine sufferer succumbs to relatively infrequent attacks, say once or twice a month, it will probably suffice for these to be treated *symptomatically* and not prophylactically. Prophylaxis, over and above the self-help measures, only becomes practicable if the rate of attacks is, say, three or four times a month, and is certainly necessary for those unfortunate enough to belong to the severer categories, which can mean as many as five attacks *per week*. Prophylactic treatment is also appropriate for women with severe, protracted menstrual migraines. The measures available to prevent attacks are twofold:

1. Treatments aimed specifically at blocking the migraine mechanism's functioning, such as drugs to combat the rise in 5HT (see Chapter 6) or to act in some other relevant manner.

2. Treatments, both drugs and other kinds, aimed more generally at decreasing emotional reactivity, such as anti-depressants or relaxation therapy.

Migraine – specific drugs

The most potent drug with specific prophylactic power in migraine attacks is *methysergide*, known also by its proprietary names of Deseril in Britain and Sansert in the USA. It is of no value during an acute attack but effective in preventing one, unlike many other frequently prescribed drugs that produce no better results than dummy tablets. Just how it works is not fully understood. It is an ergot alkaloid (with the full chemical name of lysergic acid butan-olamide) that was first used over fifteen years ago by Sicuteri (see also p. 39) who was struck by the drug's striking effects on serotonin (or 5HT), the substance released from blood platelets thought to be implicated in the neuro-vascular reactions in migraine. Methysergide 'antagonised' serotonin so effectively that for a time it was claimed to be 'the' answer to migraine for all but a few sufferers. In the event it proved to be less astounding than was at first anticipated, though perhaps as many as three-quarters of severe migraine conditions (the precise percentage is difficult to pinpoint as medical opinion varies quite widely) may be helped by its use. Certainly many doctors continue to pay tribute to its effectiveness including Arnold Friedman who, over the space of ten years, used it in over 2000 patients with vascular headaches of a migrainous nature.

However, the consensus of opinion over methysergide is, in Dr Friedman's words, that it is only appropriate for 'a limited number of patients who have failed to respond to any other type of treatment for prevention of their migraine attacks'.

Methysergide is a powerful drug in several ways. Not only does it have anti-serotonin effects, but it also acts as an anti-histamine drug as well as reducing inflammation, and it may be that these properties, alongside others, contribute largely to its effectiveness in migraine prevention. At present we simply do not know precisely how it works. But we do know for certain that it is as dangerous as it is effective, with very serious and far-reaching side-effects if not used with extreme care by doctors and patients.

The side-effects include nausea, vomiting, loss of appetite, diz-ziness, abdominal pains, skin rashes, blood disorders, weight gain, mood changes and a condition known as retro-peritoneal fibrosis which prevents one from urinating. To avoid these effects, patients taking the drug must follow rigorously their doctor's instructions, with a daily maximum dose of about 6–8 mg. These instructions will, and should, include a lay-off period of four weeks every six months or so (sometimes every four months) and will incorporate a gradual dosage increase up to the top level required. Sometimes the dosage is de-creased gradually.

Certain sorts of migraine sufferers should not take methysergide: children; pregnant women; people suffering from heart or circulatory disorders, high blood pressure, impaired kidney or liver functions or oedema (excess fluid), or peptic ulcers. Apart from these, provided strictly controlled quantities are taken, methysergide can provide (and has provided) immense relief from acute attacks. Like every drug it carries some risks to some people some of the time. Certainly doctors never use it casually or automatically, even for severe cases, while its use in milder forms of migraine is universally deplored.

Other, less powerful, anti-serotonin drugs exist. These are *BC105* (Pizotifen) which in addition checks histamine build-up. Its side-effects are drowsiness and increased appetite and body weight. Also in this category is *cyproheptidine* (Periactin) another serotonin antagonist with anti-histaminic properties that also stimulates the appetite.

Another type of drug favoured by doctors in preventing attacks is *clonidine* (trade name Dixarit in the UK, but not yet on the market in the US) which is a 'nor-adrenaline antagonist', acting on the blood vessels to make them less sensitive to amines circulating in them and hence less likely to dilate or constrict. This means that, although clonidine has relatively little impact on serotonin levels, it can bring relief especially to certain dietary migraine sufferers whose bodies cope badly with an excess of tyramine present in cheese and other foods. Initially it was developed as a drug to combat high blood pressure and has the advantage of being usable for those sufferers who also have cardiovascular disease.

Clonidine is not without side-effects, including dryness of the mouth, drowsiness, constipation, itching and swelling, sometimes nausea and dizziness. Pregnant women and those with certain arterial diseases (like Raynaud's disease) may take the drug but under the strictest possible medical supervision.

Other drugs exist for blocking the release of nor-adrenaline, such as *Indoramin* (an 'alpha receptor' blocking drug) and *propranolol* (trade name Inderal) which blocks the so-called beta-receptors. The action of these substances is to reduce the effects of stimulation brought on by stress or excitement by acting on the nerve endings (receptors) that step up the rate and force at which the heart beats. They reduce the volume of blood pumped out with each contraction of the heart and lower blood pressure. Once more, propanolol has its limitations for people with certain other conditions, e.g. pregnancy, bronchial asthma or partial heart block, and so on. Side-effects such as nausea or insomnia can occur. These drugs are, like all others used in migraine treatment, still undergoing clinical tests by researchers in various parts of the world. Until extensive tests have been carried out in controlled situations it is impossuble to say with any degree of accuracy just how effective they might be. Individual responses to drugs vary enormously. The golden rule for patient and doctor is to approach their use with qualified optimism and extreme circumspection.

Further drug approaches to prevention

Just like their historical counterparts, today's doctors are constantly trying out different sorts of drugs thought to act specifically in migraine attacks. For example, because more women than men get migraine, and therefore hormone cycles seem likely to be relevant to the issue, it has been reasoned that the hormone progesterone could be a useful measure. Progesterone is secreted naturally in the second half of the menstrual cycle when headaches are reportedly less frequent, so some doctors have attempted to imitate these conditions by progesterone injections or suppositories. The results of these attempts have been fairly mixed, with some researchers disagreeing with others about their efficacy. Again, provided strictly controlled dosages are given, progesterone therapy can be worth trying, but do not feel freakish if it does nothing to curb your headaches while your neighbour's seem to have been all but eliminated by virtually identical treatment. The same holds true for diuretics to help relieve water retention before periods. It works for some people and not for others because, to modify the words of the hymn, migraine moves in a mysterious way – and so do migraineurs' responses to drugs. This is something sufferers often quickly learn. Studies in Britain, America and Scandinavia point to the fact that women learned to adjust their own dosages of progesterone, stepping them up at times of stress or when a migraine attack seemed imminent. Conversely, women during the menopause can sometimes anticipate missing a period in one month and postpone self-administered treatment accordingly.

Non-specific measures

It is now generally accepted that in Britain (and probably elsewhere) no less than one-third of all the people consulting their family doctor are there not because of a truly physical illness but because of some kind of underlying 'emotional' or 'psychological' problem. These problems are wide ranging, from long-standing sexual difficulties to sudden out-of-the-blue depressions, and their numbers appear to be growing. According to Dr Oliver Sacks, migraine, which we know to be 'physiological' in the sense that bodily changes occur during attacks, also comes partly into this same category of a 'psychogenic' disorder; that is one with an emotional basis. He states: 'a majority of patients with extremely frequent, severe, intractable migraines are caught in a situation of severe emotional stress or conflict (of which they may or may not be aware) and ... this drives the migraine as a psychosomatic expression of their underlying emotional problems.' This point of view is not shared by all doctors. Most will recognise that stress is a component of a migraine attack but some will not subscribe to the Freudian psychoanalytical interpretation of that stress, namely that it is not just the ebb and flow of daily life that causes emotional problems but long-standing and profound conflicts at an unconscious level. Freud, incidentally, was himself a migraine sufferer.

However, whatever the nature of emotional stress, the end-product is much the same, and in recent years a number of doctors have experimented with various forms of relaxation therapy in the hope of preventing attacks. Some have pinned more faith on it than others.

Drugs

The migraineur is not 'mentally ill'. Like everyone else he is prone to bouts of worrying, sleeplessness and depression for a thousand and one everyday reasons. If attacks appear to be related to such states then numerous tranquillisers, sedatives and anti-depressants are readily available for the doctor to prescribe. Of these a well-known drug is *diazepam* (Valium) which, like all medication, must be taken in accordance with qualified medical advice. Usually the dosages are small, 2 mg two or three times a day and the beneficial effects are felt after a few weeks of starting on a controlled regimen. Valium like the other well-known minor tranquilliser Librium (chlordiazepoxide) can relieve tension but has its potentially harmful aspects. If you have severe headaches, taking a larger than normal dose of valium will have a pronounced sedative effect but this drowsiness will not necessarily reduce the number and severity of the headaches. Other drugs in this category are *amylobarbitone*, *phenytoin*, *amitriptyline* and *imipramine*, all of which are packaged under a number of trade names. Their effects are to relax tension or lift depression but, in excess, they all have adverse effects of various kinds. Certain categories of sufferers such as pregnant women or people with heart disorders must always approach these drugs with extreme care. None of them is suitable for taking casually or carelessly, however bad the headache, because many have effects that are not yet fully understood.

One category of anti-depressant is very definitely to be avoided by all migraine sufferers who have a strong predisposition towards tyramine excess as a precipitating factor (see Chapter 8). These are the *monoamine oxidase inhibitors* (MAOIs) which not only act to relieve depression but also, as their name implies, affect the breakdown of amines, including substances like tyramine in cheese. So taking these drugs (which anyway are losing favour among doctors for various other reasons) may help to alleviate your depression but not, in the process, eliminate attacks.

Relaxation therapy

As well as drugs, it is often suggested that tense patients would benefit from various kinds of psychotherapy to help them cope with emotional problems and conflicts. Be that as it may, there seem to have been very few attempts to provide this specifically for headache sufferers. On the other hand, general relaxation therapy has been tried out and, reportedly, improved the lot of some sufferers.

Relaxation techniques for helping to cope with physical illness are not new. Edmund Jacobson was using them in America in the 1930s when he studied the effect of mental activities on muscle tension. He found that if a person is relaxed his muscles register a slightly different electrical potential to the contracted, tense state. On this basis he got a number of patients to try to recognise the degree of muscle tensions in their bodies and to control this tension. Muscle tension, a feeling of tightness round the head, is well known to migraine sufferers. Most of them have scalp muscle tension headaches as well as migraine and this often shows in rigidity of posture, clenching of hands and even perhaps grinding of teeth during sleep.

In such circumstances, fatigue builds up which again can lay the sufferer open to attack. So relaxation would seem to be a possible route towards alleviating the situation. In order to test out some of Jacobson's ideas on migraine sufferers (though they have been used in other contexts as well, from childbirth to preparing athletes for major events), Hay and Madders did a long-term study into the effects of group relaxation therapy using patients referred to them by a specialist clinic or their own doctors. All the sufferers had severe

disabling attacks, usually two or more per month and lasting one day
or longer. Furthermore they had not responded to some of the
routine pharmacological treatments outlined above. In all, ninety-
eight patients attended a series of six evening sessions of relaxation
training, consisting of exercises followed by group discussion. The
results were as follows:

No. of Patients	Progress
69	Less frequent, less severe or shorter attacks
25	No change
4	Attacks were worse
98	

What training did the classes give? Below are some extracts from an
article published by Hay and Madders in the *Journal of the Royal
College of General Practitioners* in which they described their results:

Throughout the classes patients work in pairs, changing partners
at intervals in order to feel the difference in a contracted muscle
and a relaxed one. Experience has shown that this is a most effective way of recognising skeletal muscle tension, but an added benefit is the rapport established with other members when physical
contact and friendly discussion is involved.

Simple swinging movements appear to be the most successful
method of inducing relaxation in arms. Relaxation of neck, shoulder and facial muscles is practised sitting on chairs with a partner
standing behind and assisting with contrasted tension and relaxation. Firm, gentle smoothing of the forehead assists in reducing
tension around the eyes. It is in this region that the most marked
anxiety inhibiting effects are usually obtained and a calmer and
more tranquil expression is observed.

Relaxation of other parts of the body is followed by a period of
deep relaxation lying on blankets on the floor. Relaxation is
preceded by regular deep abdominal breathing with the emphasis
on expiration and 'letting go'. (Patients frequently report difficulty
and guilt feeling at letting tension go.) At all times it is emphasised
that relaxation is a conscious active process under the direct control of the patient. Imagery is discouraged and patients are not
expected to sleep during the class. Support by way of verbal

instructions is gradually diminished so that by the final session patients go through the procedure on their own.

At each session attention is drawn to the use of muscle relaxation in everyday life; relaxation of shoulders when driving, typing, sitting; relaxation of face and shoulders combined with deep breathing at times of stress; a short spell of horizontal relaxation after work and before the evening meal and general relaxation before sleep and if wakened in the night.

The exercise session is followed by refreshments and discussion in small groups of five or six. Patients are invited to talk about their symptoms and share their experiences and we recognise that this is in direct contrast to their experience of boring their relatives and friends. They are told that this information is valuable for the purpose of the investigation. The groups have no acknowledged leader but as questions are raised answers are given to the whole class. At one session the general-practitioner consultant from the migraine clinic attends and joins in the discussion. Patients talk freely and discussions are lively, thoughtful and sometimes hilarious. As the course progresses emphasis is shifted towards discussion of the effects and practice methods of relaxation.

At the fifth session past members are invited to join the class for a refresher session and their success has been encouraging to new members. At the final session relatives or friends are invited to observe or join in so that they can give support and understanding to home practice.

The initial finding that this kind of programme *could* help migraine sufferers has been borne out by later research. Interestingly, too, nearly three-quarters of the people attending these classes (in Birmingham) not only said that their attacks had become less severe, they also reported that they had been able to reduce their dependence on medicines, some to the extent of doing without them altogether.

Is relaxation therapy as useful as it appears to be from these classes? Certainly it does help one to understand one's bodily reactions better and does not involve complicated postures or meditation that some people find difficult or undesirable. On the other hand, relaxation helps those who are most strongly inclined to help themselves. It is probably not suitable for those people who are heavily dependent on drugs, say, for severe depression. These particular classes were held on a group basis and sufferers had the added bonus of being able to swap experiences. If you hate group activities of any kind, your ability to relax would be severely limited. If you do fall into this category, bear in mind that the real value of relaxation therapy is not what is done in class but at home, day in day out, and there are a number of books, records and tapes available to help you to practise. Here are a few pointers to relaxation at home:

(a) Try to recognise muscle tension throughout the day, especially on those occasions when you are ostensibly relaxing in an easy chair. Is the chair really comfortable? Does it provide support for the back, shoulders and thighs? Are you tensing muscles in the neck or shoulders or stomach?

(b) Preface any relaxation exercise with a short period of deep breathing, being calm and deliberate about breathing out.

(c) Try to organise at least one short period in the day for a time of complete relaxation as opposed to the partial relaxation you can achieve all the time by greater awareness of the body's tension. Let the mind relax too, drifting along and even dropping off into a short nap if the mood takes you.

(d) Relaxation comes from self-awareness. Don't opt for strenuous exercise to induce exhaustion but choose the measured, breathing-related programmes that are easy to practise at any time and unpartnered.

(e) Cultivate a technique for 'unlocking' the body's muscles. Lie down comfortably in a quiet room. Begin with one arm. Sense and tense each upper arm muscle, then let it go limp. Do the same with the lower arm, the hand, then the fingers. Then move on to the other arm, followed by the rest of the body, legs, neck, abdomen and so on. Think about the facial muscles, the forehead, eyes and cheeks and in turn get them to go limp.

'Learning to relax' is not that easy for some people. You are trying to let go of something and in trying you can defeat the purpose. So take your time.

You may feel that some of the meditative approaches to relaxation would work for you, or perhaps Yoga. If so, by all means try them out, and try not to get discouraged if at first they do not seem to help. You will need time to become proficient.

Biofeedback

As a sort of electronically-based extension of relaxation training, biofeedback may have something positive to offer the sufferer. Certainly some people are, albeit tenatively, claiming that it does. Biofeedback is a technique for 'feeding back' information about a person's bodily functions to that person using a visual display. It can show heart rate by means of a light, a red light, say, for a normal rate and a green one for a slower-than-normal rate, etc. Once the person has learnt to discriminate between various physiological states (normal fast, slow, and so on) then the way is clear to learning to control them. That is the theory of biofeedback, though just *how* a person can learn to control his physiological responses is far from clear; it is a skill akin to the self-control attained by monks or gurus in the course of transcendental meditation, which sometimes reaches astonishing levels. Quite by chance, biofeedback was applied to migraine research when some workers at the Menninger Foundation Clinic suggested that skin temperature biofeedback could help to abort migraine attacks. Accordingly experiments were done with six migraine sufferers who were hooked up to the biofeedback machinery and given a display of their hand temperatures. They were then asked to sit and think about making their hands hotter, and sure enough they all managed to raise the temperatures accordingly. Then they were asked to do this themselves whenever they felt attacks coming on; and, amazingly, by increasing hand temperatures they were able to reduce the number and intensity of attacks. Just why and how they were able to do this is still not clear. Perhaps biofeedback in some way helped them to branch into their sympathetic nervous system's activity; perhaps it was a 'relaxation response'; an increase in self-control; or a redistribution of blood. Or perhaps a combination of all of these. Whatever the reasons, quite a few respectable university psychologists throughout the world are sanguine about the potential for biofeedback, though as yet there have been too few trials with headache sufferers for any to be conclusive. As with relaxation, biofeedback is an active form of therapy on the part of the sufferer. He or she has to want to learn the skills involved, and concentrate very hard to apply them successfully. At present this is not a universally available treatment, being very much at the experimental stage, but it is likely to grow in popularity, perhaps very rapidly. Certainly there will be no shortage of volunteers.

Other preventive measures
Another technique which has recently come into some prominence is

the old Chinese art/science of acupuncture which uses needles placed in various, seemingly unconnected, sites of the body in order to readjust its malfunctioning. To Western doctors, the idea of repairing or relieving a diseased organ by methods such as acupuncture that are based not on scientific method but on philosophical speculation is quite alien. On the other hand, some non-Chinese doctors are beginning to try out acupuncture and reporting favourably on its effects. So far as migraine is concerned there is no evidence available to influence the sufferer one way or another. If you want to try acupuncture, do so. If it works, it works. The same is true of another fairly controversial technique, hypnosis, which has also been offered as a migraine 'cure'.

Hypnosis is really an extreme form of suggestion in which the person being hypnotised is required to surrender himself temporarily to the hypnotist. This can only take place within certain limits and is not as unsavoury as lurid films and books would have us believe. On the other hand, suggestibility varies considerably between individuals and not all attempts to induce hypnotic trances are successful. When they are, the state of consciousness produced can be used to advantage by some practitioners who claim to have helped neurotic patients to overcome their problems. Can hypnosis help the migraineur? It *may* help him or her to relax more in everyday life, *if* conditions for hypnosis are right and the sufferer is totally co-operative. But beyond that there is no evidence that hypnosis can 'prevent' migraine. It is a tool not a panacea.

Hypnosis and techniques such as chiropractic treatment (backbone manipulation) are all fringe medical practices that your family doctor may know of but, in the vast majority of cases, will not be able to employ himself. There are 'justifications' in all of them for applying them to migraine, some more convincing than others. If you are seriously thinking of undergoing a course of treatment with a practitioner of one of these methods, talk to your doctor first about some of the potential side-effects and/or hazards.

Lastly, there is the most drastic prophylaxis of all, surgery. Since migraine is a disorder of function not of structure – between attacks the body is perfectly normal – there is little argument for interfering with its structure by removing teeth, tonsils or gall-bladder (all of which have been carried out in the past). In particular, it is a myth for women to believe in hysterectomy as a permanent cure. Removing the ovaries can be followed by a period of relief but the attacks are likely to re-establish themselves later on in an identical or different pattern. Surgical intervention will do nothing for the migraine sufferer except perhaps fulfil some deep masochistic need to be operated on in order to get better. Even more specific surgery, such as that done on the nerves of the temporal artery in the case of severe one-sided migraine, seems to be of questionable value and is best avoided because any relief it brings seems to be very short-lived.

13

Research, Clinics and Activities
Worldwide

'. . . *the invisible pressure of thousands and thousands of migraine
sufferers, all crying "Help me, Help me!"* '
                                    Pamela Hansford Johnson

Treating migraine, as we saw in earlier chapters, is both a specialist
and a non-specialist matter. Each individual sufferer, regardless of
how much he knows about medicine, is to some extent able to frame
his way of living to meet his problem nearly halfway. Together with a
general practitioner one should arrive at a satisfactory long-term
method of reducing and alleviating attacks, using some of the various
techniques described in this book.

On the other hand, there is a body of doctors, usually though not
invariably neurologists, for whom migraine work is a specialist
activity, both in terms of providing treatment and in researching into
causes and possible cures. Their treatment and research go hand in
hand because, working as they often do in specialist clinics, they have
a chance to see sufferers during or even just before acute attacks
(unlike the general practitioner who can do so infrequently) and
thereby observe some of the vascular and biochemical phenomena
known to be taking place as they are happening.

Specialised migraine clinics are relatively new, but quite well
established now as a feature of hospital out-patient departments in
big cities. In Britain the Migraine Trust (founded in 1965) started in
1971 the City Migraine Clinic in London, later to become the
Princess Margaret Clinic, which in the first five years of operation
saw over 6000 patients referred by their family doctors and gave
treatment for 2000 acute headaches during attacks. When one thousand of these patients were studied it was found that women outnum-
bered men by nearly two to one; that one-third had classical symptoms, one-third common migraine while of the rest the majority had

'tension' headaches. The Director of the Clinic, Dr Marcia Wilkinson, and her team provide not only a range of treatments for patients but also carry out a research programme that is of considerable importance. So successful has this clinic been that it has acted as a model for others in Britain and elsewhere. At the Charing Cross Hospital in London there is a similar specialist unit directed by Dr F. Clifford Rose which has, since its opening a few years ago, also proved both that there is strong demand for such services and that they are effective in times of acute need. Most people's headaches have improved by the time they leave the clinic (though they still complain of 'grogginess' or 'sore heads'), and they generally feel 'better in themselves' and more confident about coping in the future.

In America there are some specialist clinics and doctors, numerically fairly few considering the size of the US migraine problem, but certainly showing signs of expansion. According to one such specialist Dr John R. Graham, Director of the Headache Research Foundation in Boston, there is a difference in emphasis in the way the two countries tackle migraine treatment. He points out that in Britain a clinic like the Princess Margaret seems to get the same or even better results than its American counterparts with smaller amounts of medicine being given to patients. Instead of trying to prepare the incoming sufferers to get back quickly to their place of work, the British approach is to provide a more peaceful climate – an atmosphere of 'flight not fight'. He says of fellow American doctors 'we tend to use more medicine in an effort to keep people going, maybe we should be taking more steps towards making them stop or slow down.'

Research

It is not (yet) known what 'causes' migraine nor whether it will indeed ever yield to a definitive 'cure' even though so far a good deal of research energy and resources have been expended in trying to find out. There is, however, no doubt at all that positive though limited advances have been made in recent years both in our understanding of the mechanism of migraine and how to relieve its effects, not enough perhaps to bring unqualified solace to the acute sufferer but certainly more than many people, sufferers included, probably realise. It is also certain that, in the future, migraine research must be of an integrated kind. One definition of the condition describes it as a 'genetically anchored, mentally conditioned, neurally conveyed and humorally affected paroxysmal, vascular disorder'. If this is so – and few people would dispute it – then researchers are faced with the need to orchestrate their work to take in genetics, psychology, neurology, biochemistry, psychiatry, serology, pharmacology and quite a few other 'ologies'. The following are the main directions this multi-disciplinary research is like to take.

1. Empirical work with existing tools

Everyday work at places like the migraine clinics involves trying combinations of existing drugs and developing preventive measures such as relaxation therapy and avoidance of possible precipitants. This is, in part, directly for helping patients, in part experimental, and it is research of this kind that is especially valuable not least because clinics have such large numbers of migrainous subjects to study. The one drawback to this sort of research is the nature of the samples it uses. By definition, people who go to doctors and attend clinics are a persistent and unrepresentative minority, a self-selected group that may give the researchers studying them false ideas about migraine and migraineurs in general. There is a continuing need for trying to broaden out such studies of established treatments and their effectiveness to include more reference to the general migraine population.

2. Clinical trials of new drugs – a money problem

If a pharmaceutical company develops a new drug for migraine, whether this be a pain reliever, prophylactic or some other preparation, it has to carry out various tests before it can, legally, confidently launch its product on to the market. One test is for possible harmful effects, toxicity, which can be carried out using laboratory animals. But, once the toxicity hurdle is overcome, the drug then has to be tested on humans to see whether it is effective and, if it is, what dosage levels are required. Migraine clinics are ideally placed to carry out tests of this kind because they can choose from among their many patients those who are best suited to act as experimental subjects, screening out those who are unsuitable on grounds of general health, age, nature and frequency of attacks, and so on. Sometimes these tests are 'open' or pilot trials in which patients are given the drug under scrutiny and asked to comment on its effectiveness. Sometimes the researchers use a technique called 'double blind' trials in which both genuine and dummy (placebo) tablets are administered, with neither doctor nor patient knowing which is which, so that any comments on the effectiveness of the medicine will not be prejudiced in favour of (or against) a product for one reason or another. Many people – and not only migraine sufferers – say that they 'feel better' whatever they are given, provided they believe that it is something 'new'. The fact that it may be just the novelty and not the pharmacological action of the tablets or suppositories that is achieving results is, of course, of considerable importance for all concerned.

Testing new drugs is, therefore, a complicated and often long-drawn-out process. Added to this, migraine is proving still to be a particularly resilient nut to crack, and pharmaceutical companies (on whom much of the research burden must fall) are becoming more and more reluctant to invest huge sums in what could turn out to be abortive lines of enquiry. The drug clonidine used as a means of reducing the migraineur's blood vessel sensitivity was originally developed to combat hypertension; its usefulness in migraine only emerged later. Drug companies are less likely to spend £5–10 million on fundamental research into migraine itself, only to find themselves in another blind alley. Their potential rewards, if, say, a new super-efficient prophylactic tablet could be developed, would be prodigious but, seen as a business venture, such research looks highly speculative.

3. Statistical research

Another important line of enquiry for researchers is to survey groups of people to find out about the prevalence of migraine and such epidemiological matters as to whether certain occupations or social circumstances give rise to it more than others. This kind of statistical work needs to draw on data collected from large groups of people or to garner information from carefully selected samples. It is difficult research to do properly, employing sophisticated methods of data collection and processing, but, done with great care, it can produce valuable results. Factors such as the geographical distribution of migraine can be looked at in relation to innumerable possible causative factors ranging from density of population to climatic conditions, all these being processed by computer for the researcher to interpret. Again, data provided by sufferers is vital, especially in providing follow-up information on aspects such as the decline of attacks with age, pregnancy, contraception, and so on. So far as the migraine sufferer is concerned, co-operating on surveys of this kind is one positive way of helping to beat migraine; good personal note-taking is, anyway, a valuable aid to avoiding precipitating factors, so why not let it be doubly valuable in ultimately helping fellow-sufferers?

4. Causes

A good deal of research into the causes of migraine concerns itself with the action of the blood vessels and how their constriction or expansion relates to the progress of an attack. This sort of work involves many types of studies: cerebral blood flow; arterial calibre changes; blood composition and chemical changes are all relevant in migraine and are being scrutinised from all sorts of angles using a battery of techniques. The same holds true for brain cell activity which EEGs investigate using electrodes placed on special points on the scalp which are wired to a recording device. An example of EEG research is that done on light response. In these experiments lights are flashed before the eyes of people connected up to the machine and the electrical events in their brains studied with a view to determining how different conditions evoke different responses. From this it may be possible to say something about the migraineur's particular sensitivity to bright, dazzling lights which can act as a trigger for attacks, or about his dislike of light (photophobia) while a migraine is in progress.

Such biological activities as hormonal fluctuations are clearly implicated in migraine, not to mention the role of allergic responses in modifying the individual's 'migraine threshold' or the importance of certain amines in our food. All these fields have been opened up and scientists are constantly learning more about even fairly basic aspects of them. Progress has been made and will continue to be made – provided sufficient funds are available – but often in tiny steps at a time, some seemingly trivial but each contributing to the whole.

Organisations

Just as research into migraine needs co-ordination of the various branches of science involved in its study, so internationally there is a burning need for a strong co-ordinated umbrella organisation. Throughout the world, and especially in industrialised countries, stress and stress-related illnesses are on the increase, as the upward trend of figures for heart disorder all too clearly show. Migraine, too, appears to be on the increase but, unfortunately, there is at present no 'World Migraine Federation' to meet this challenge with a united front, no universally-available front-line treatment such as the specialist clinics can provide for a lucky few; no vast international network of freely-exchanged blood or urine samples for researchers to study at will.

Nevertheless, awareness of migraine is growing. In Britain there are now two organisations, the Migraine Trust which is the sponsor and co-ordinator of much research in the field, as well as an invaluable source of information, encouragement, advice and training; and the British Migraine Association which is basically a sufferers' group publishing (as does the Trust) its own newsletter and many other useful items such as Ernest Burd's clearly-written leaflet on self-help relaxation treatment. In America there are two organisations: the American Association for the Study of Headache, a body of 350 doctors specialising in the subject and publishing the journal *Headache* (the UK counterpart to this is *Hemicrania* which ceased publication in 1976); and the National Migraine Foundation, a fairly young volunteer group for sufferers. It, too, publishes a highly readable newsletter. Parallel organisations exist in other parts of the world, including Scandinavia, Canada and Australia, though the degree of centralisation varies considerably. As an indication of the rising tide of interest, an international symposium sponsored by the British Migraine Trust attracted some 250 experts drawn from no fewer than thirty countries.

Some addresses

UK

The Migraine Trust, 45 Great Ormond Street, London WC1

British Migraine Association, Evergreen, Ottermead Lane, Ottershaw, Chertsey, Surrey KT16 0HJ

Princess Margaret Migraine Clinic, 22 Charterhouse Street, London EC1

Charing Cross Migraine Clinic

USA

American Association for the Study of Headache, 5252 N Western Avenue, Chicago, Illinois 60625

National Migraine Foundation, 2422 W Foster Avenue, Chicago, Illinois 60625

California Medical Clinic for Headache, 16542 Ventura Boulevard, Encino, CA 91316

Diamond Headache Clinic Ltd, 5252 N Western Avenue, Chicago, Illinois 60625

Mt Sinai Hospital Medical Center, 5th Avenue and 100th, New York, NY 10029

Southwest Headache Group, 6036 North 19th Avenue, Suite 205, Phoenix, AZ 85015

University of Kansas Medical Center, Department of Medicine, Kansas City, KS 66103

AUSTRALIA

Division of Neurology, Prince Henry Hospital, Sydney

NEW ZEALAND

Department of Medicine Clinical School, Wellington Hospital, Wellington 2, New Zealand

CANADA

The Migraine Foundation, 390 Brunswick Avenue, Toronto, Ontario M5R 2Z4

14

Perspectives

If the stubbornly complicated nature of migraine continues to confuse you, this is hardly surprising. It has confused the medical world for centuries and seems likely to go on for a while eluding capture. In the past few decades perhaps as many as four hundred remedies have been put forward, some to the accompaniment of enormous enthusiasm, only to be for the most part thrown on the pharmaceutical scrap heap, leaving almost as much puzzlement as before. However, little by little understanding continues to grow, while treatments are based more and more often on carefully controlled, objective studies. At the same time, trial and error still persist among desperate patients, often with some success. One sufferer, a butcher by trade, discovered that he could cure his attacks by spending a short spell in his walk-in freezer. Long may he continue to help himself in this way. If you feel better by wearing a string of beads or doing transcendental meditation or having your hair cut short, then by all means do whatever helps you. You are discovering the power of the placebo effect that doctors have known about ever since the first prescription was dispensed. It may be mumbo-jumbo rather than medical science but, at the end of the day, who cares?

Many people are finding out that certain preventive measures can work for them and that carefully regulated treatments in attacks are genuinely helpful. If the sufferer is to give these measures the best possible chance of working, some effort is undoubtedly required on his own part. Possible precipitants *must* be noted down; treatment regimens involving drugs, even common ones like aspirin, *must* be adhered to scrupulously; and in general unnecessary stresses and strains of everyday living avoided.

Despite these precautions many sufferers remain miserable and unconvinced of the usefulness of their doctor in helping them with their migraine. Sometimes they have just cause to be dissatisfied because their general practitioner may be too overloaded (or too uninterested in the condition) to be of much use. In cases like this, the sufferer should seek a second opinion, shop around until demand and supply are properly in phase. Sometimes of course it is the general practitioner who takes the initiative, referring the migraineur to a specialist for help. Perhaps he (the GP) is unsure of his diagnosis, perhaps the diagnosis was accurate but the treatment he has been trying inappropriate, perhaps he is simply tired of his protracted and unsatisfactory dealings with a particular patient. Some sufferers insist, despite all reassurances to the contrary, that their headaches must be the pains of a malignant brain tumour and they need to be told afresh by a third party that this is not so. Others latch on to firm notions about treatment that are not acceptable to some doctors but could be employed by others, in which case why not change?

Having established a satisfactory relationship with your doctor it is as well to retain a cautious optimism towards the whole business of treatment. One doctor put this as follows: 'Learn to *accept* that the occasional attack may continue, but that usually within 24–48 hours you will be well again. If this attitude is achieved migraine can be regarded as an occasional if very unpleasant nuisance.' If you are in good general health, apart from the migraines, you may even count yourself lucky that these are the only thing that bother you, or even that in some curious way they act as a sort of alternative to other perhaps more serious complaints. This is an understandable attitude and one that some doctors have subscribed to. They have characterised the migraineur as a person who, if he did not have his attacks, might well be prone to all manner of other ailments. This is a bit like the myth that babies who cry a lot are particularly intelligent. There is no evidence for this but it is a crumb of consolation perhaps for the parent roused from sleep by an infant's cries in the middle of the night. No, migraine does not confer immunity from other illnesses nor, conversely, does it make one more susceptible to them. To paraphrase the old Jewish joke: 'Migraine sufferers and Jews are just like everyone else. Only more so!'

Further Reading

Background to migraine, Proceedings of the Symposia sponsored by the Migraine Trust. Volumes 1–5 (1966, 1967, 1969, 1970, 1972) published by Heinemann. Volumes 6–7 (1974, 1976) available from the Migraine Trust

Diamond, Seymour and Furlong, William, *More than two aspirin*, Follett Publishing, 1976

Freese, Arthur, *Headaches, the kinds and the cures*, Allen and Unwin, 1976

Hanington, Edda, *Migraine*, Priory Press, 1974

Hay, K. M., *Do something about that migraine*, 1968

McQuade, Walter and Aikman, Ann, *Stress, how to stop your mind killing your body*, Hutchinson, 1976

Migraine, mystery and misery, published by the Migraine Trust

Office of Health Economics, *Migraine*, OHE Paper No. 41, 1972

Rachman, S. J. and Philips, Clare, *Psychology and medicine*, Temple Smith, 1975

Ritchie Russell, W., *Explaining the brain*, Oxford University Press, 1975

Sacks, Oliver W., *Migraine, the evolution of a common disorder*, Faber, 1970

Saxena, Pramod (ed.), *Migraine and related headaches*, Sandoz, 1974

Waters, W. E., *The epidemiology of migraine*, Boehringer Ingelheim, 1974

Wilkinson, Marcia, *Living with migraine*, Heinemann, 1976

Wolff, H. G., *Headache and other head pain*, Oxford University Press, 1963

Index